Nurse Aide Exam
Review Cards

Barbara Acello, MS, RN

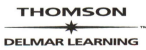

THOMSON
★
DELMAR LEARNING

Australia Canada Mexico Singapore Spain United Kingdom United States

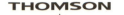

THOMSON

DELMAR LEARNING

Nurse Aide Exam Review Cards
by Barbara Acello, MS, RN

Executive Director Health Care
Business Unit:
William Brotmiller

Executive Editor:
Cathy L. Esperti

Acquisitions Editor:
Sherry Gomoll

Technology Project Manager:
Joseph Saba

Executive Marketing Manager:
Dawn F. Gerrain

Art/Design Coordinator:
Connie Lundberg-Watkins

Project Editor:
Bryan Viggiani

Production Coordinator:
Catherine Ciardullo

Editorial Assistant:
Jennifer Conklin

Printed in the United States of America
1 2 3 4 5 XXX 05 04 03 02

For more information contact Delmar Learning,
5 Maxwell Drive
Clifton Park, NY 12065-2919

Or find us on the World Wide Web at http://www.delmar.com

For permission to use material from this text or product, contact us by
Tel (800) 730-2214
Fax (800) 730-2215
www.thomsonrights.com

Library of Congress Cataloging-in-Publication Data

ISBN 1401808336 Package 140180831X

NOTICE TO THE READER

Publisher does not warrant or guarantee any of the products described herein or perform any independent analysis in connection with any of the product information contained herein. Publisher does not assume, and expressly disclaims, any obligation to obtain and include information other than that provided to it by the manufacturer.

The reader is expressly warned to consider and adopt all safety precautions that might be indicated by the activities herein and to avoid all potential hazards. By following the instructions contained herein, the reader willingly assumes all risks in connection with such instructions.

The Publisher makes no representation or warranties of any kind, including but not limited to, the warranties of fitness for particular purpose or merchantability, nor are any such representations implied with respect to the material set forth herein, and the publisher takes no responsibility with respect to such material. The publisher shall not be liable for any special, consequential, or exemplary damages resulting, in whole or part, from the readers' use of, or reliance upon, this material.

Contents

Introduction

Review Cards

Activities of Daily Living: Hygiene

Activities of Daily Living: Dressing and Grooming

Activities of Daily Living: Nutrition and Hydration

Activities of Daily Living: Elimination

Activities of Daily Living: Rest/Comfort/Sleep

Basic Nursing Skills: Infection Control

Basic Nursing Skills: Safety/Emergency

Basic Nursing Skills: Therapeutic/Technical Procedures

Basic Nursing Skills: Data Collection and Reporting

Restorative Services: Prevention

Restorative Services: Self Care/Independence

Psychosocial Care Skills: Emotional and Mental Health Needs

Psychosocial Care Skills: Spiritual and Cultural Needs

Role of the Nurse Aide: Communication

Role of the Nurse Aide: Client Rights

Role of the Nurse Aide: Legal and Ethical Behavior

Role of the Nurse Aide: Member of the Health Care Team

Notes

Acknowledgments

A special thank you to all the reviewers who offered many wonderful suggestions:

Jodi Badgley, RN, BA
Lee County High Tech Center North
Cape Coral, FL

Beverly Boyd, RN
Grand River Voc-Tech School
Chillicothe, MO

CJ Gilberte, RN, BS, HCM
Tri-Cities ROP
Whittier CA

Catherine Johnson, LVN
Innovations in Health Care
El Paso, TX

Introduction

Nurse Aide Written Test Overview

The nurse aide written test covers the main content areas that you studied in class. These are:

- Physical Care Skills
    - ❖ Activities of daily living (ADLs)
        - ■ hygiene
        - ■ dressing and grooming
        - ■ nutrition and hydration
        - ■ elimination
        - ■ comfort, rest, and sleep
- Basic Nursing Skills
    - ■ infection control
    - ■ safety and emergency procedures
    - ■ therapeutic and technical procedures, such as bedmaking, specimen collection, height and weight measurement, and use of restraints
    - ■ observation, reporting, and data collection
- Restorative Nursing Care Skills
    - ■ preventive health care, such as contracture and pressure ulcer prevention
    - ■ promoting client self-care and independence
- Psychosocial Care Skills
    - ❖ Emotional and mental health needs
        - ■ behavior management
        - ■ dying clients' needs
        - ■ sexuality needs
        - ■ cultural and spiritual needs
- Role of the Nursing Assistant
    - ❖ Communication
        - ■ verbal communication
        - ■ nonverbal communication
        - ■ listening
        - ■ clients with special communication problems
    - ❖ Resident rights
    - ❖ Legal and ethical behavior
    - ❖ Responsibilities as a member of the health care team
    - ❖ Knowledge of medical terminology and abbreviations

The written state test is designed to ensure that you have the knowledge necessary to function safely as an entry-level nurse aide. The test varies in each state. In most states, the test uses between 50 and 120 questions. You will be given approximately two to four hours to complete this part of the test, depending on the number of questions your state uses. The time allowed is fairly generous. You must be on time to take the state test. Most states have a list of supplies or identification that you must bring to be admitted to the test. If you are late or fail to bring the required identification or supplies, you may not be admitted, so follow directions carefully. The test examiner will call "Time" near the end of the test to warn you that the end of the allotted time is near.

The written test questions are all in multiple-choice format, like the examples listed on your study cards. These cards use the term nurse aide to describe the individual giving care. The word client is used to describe the individual receiving care. However, various other terms may be used to describe the caregiver. These include nurse assistant and nursing assistant. Other terms that may be used to describe the person receiving care include patient and resident. Your examiner will tell you which terms are used for these individuals on your state test.

The questions on these cards are grouped by content (subject) area. However, the questions on your state test will be written randomly and will not be grouped by subject.

Many states have a practice test and candidate handbook available. Ask your instructor if these tools are available in your state. They will be invaluable in preparing for your state test. Many of the standard state tests are online at http://www.asisvcs.com. Many state nurse aide registries also maintain Web sites. If your state registry is online, you may wish to check its Web site for information about the state test.

Study Skills

No matter what type of test you take, you must first master the material. Using your index cards is an excellent way to do this. You may wish to prepare additional cards listing vocabulary terms, abbreviations, or questions from your workbook or text.

To study, look at the front of the card, and try to remember what is written on the back. Turn the card over to see if you are correct. After going through all the cards once, you may wish to shuffle them and review them again. You must be sure that you know the information in any order.

As you review the cards, begin to sort them into two piles. One pile will be for material you know well and the other pile will be for material that you are having trouble remembering. Once you have two piles, try to learn the most difficult information. Continue reviewing the cards until you have mastered the material. Review the cards several times a day during the time before the exam.

There are a number of advantages to using the card system. First, sorting the cards and preparing extra cards is a good learning experience. Second, the cards are easy and convenient to carry with you. You can study them during spare moments throughout the day. Another advantage is that you can use the cards with a friend to quiz each other.

Other Helpful Study Skills

1. Control your environment. Do whatever it takes to find a quiet place to study. Get up early in the morning, when everyone else is asleep, or find a quiet corner of the library.

2. Block out a specific time for study. Study your biorhythms to find out what time of day you function at your peak level of performance.

3. Become part of a small, dedicated study group of three to five people, or find a study partner.

4. Tackle difficult concepts first, before you get tired.

5. Get plenty of sleep.

6. Eat right, especially protein and complex carbohydrates.

7. Study key concepts by asking yourself, "What are four different ways this concept could be tested?"

8. Study all of the information included in the rationale on your study cards. Ask yourself how the information could be tested. Make sure you can apply the principles given here to similar situations.

Taking the Test

To do well on a test, you should be at your best when you start. Eat a good breakfast or lunch. Try to avoid anything that will cause stress. Leave for the test site early enough to arrive on time. Allow a little extra time for minor delays. Take a watch and two or three Number 2, sharpened, black-lead pencils with erasers. You will probably need to bring a photograph or signature identification card to show the examiner. Some states require two different forms of identification.

When you arrive at the test site, do not let another person's last-minute questions or comments upset you. Follow these general rules for taking the test:

1. You will be given verbal instructions and will be asked to complete an information form. Pay close attention to the examiner's instructions. He or she may be required to read the directions. The examiner may not be permitted to answer questions.

2. Take several deep breaths and try to relax. If you become anxious during the test, close your eyes for a few seconds and practice slow, deep breathing. Remind yourself that you have studied well and are prepared to take the test. Think positive.

3. When you receive your test booklet, review the written directions and look at any sample questions. Make sure you understand how to mark your answers. Follow directions carefully. Most state tests are computer scored, and stray marks can cause otherwise correct answers to be marked wrong.

4. Work at a steady pace.

5. Take the questions at face value. Do not read anything into the question. Avoid thinking, "What if?" Answer the question based on the information given. Do not look for trick questions or hidden meanings.

6. Read the stem of the question. Think of the answer in your own words before reading the answers. Then read all the answers given. Search for the correct alternative.

7. It may be helpful to cross out unnecessary words in the question. Distracting information has been crossed out in this example:

Q. A client who wears a wig understands that the nurse aide will not talk about this information outside the facility because this information is:

   a. legal.

   b. confidential.

   c. negligent.

   d. cultural.

8. If you do not know the answer to a question, circle the number and move on. Come back to it later. You may remember the answer later, or may find a clue to the answer in another question.

9. Be alert to words such as *not* and *except* that may completely change the intent of the question. Pay close attention to words that are *italicized*, CAPITALIZED, or are within "quotation marks" or (parentheses). These words are usually important.

10. Avoid unfamiliar choices. Information that you are unfamiliar with is probably incorrect.

11. If you don't know the answer, try to determine what it is not. Cross out answers that you know or think are incorrect. If you have crossed out two answers, you have a 50% chance of guessing correctly.

12. Look at the shortest and longest of the remaining answers. The correct answer may be shorter or longer than the others.

13. There is no penalty for guessing. If you cannot figure out the answer, it is better to guess than to leave an item blank.

14. Do not become upset if some individuals finish the test early and get up to leave. Some people read faster than others. Studies have shown that those who finish first do not necessarily get the best scores.

15. When you get to the end of the test, go back and complete any items you skipped.

16. Do not change your answers without a good reason.

17. Before turning the test in, check it to make sure you marked every answer.

Taking a Multiple Choice Test

Most standardized tests use multiple-choice items. This is because multiple-choice items can measure a variety of learning outcomes, from simple to complex. They also provide the most consistent results. The multiple-choice item consists of a stem, which presents a problem situation, and four possible choices called alternatives. The alternatives include the correct answer and several wrong answers called distractors. The stem may be a question or incomplete statement, as in this example:

- Question form:

   Q. Which of the following people is responsible for taking care of a client?
   a. janitor
   b. cook
   c. nurse aide
   d. dishwasher

- Incomplete statement form:

   Q. The care of a client is the responsibility of a:
   a. janitor
   b. cook
   c. nurse aide
   d. dishwasher

Although worded differently, both stems present the same problem. The alternatives in the examples contain only one correct answer. All distractors are clearly incorrect.

Another type of multiple-choice item is the best-answer format. In this form, the alternatives may be partially correct, but one is clearly better than the others. Look at the following example:

- Best-answer form:

   Q. Which of the following ethical behaviors is the MOST important?
   a. Maintain a positive attitude.
   b. Act as a responsible employee.
   c. Be courteous to visitors.
   d. Promote quality of life for each client.

Other variations of the best-answer form may ask you, "What is the first thing to do," the "most helpful action," the "best response or best answer," or a similar kind of question. Whether the correct answer or best-answer form is used depends on the information given.

The examples use four alternatives. The chance of guessing correctly is only one in four or 25%. Each test question has only one correct answer. Do not mark more than one answer per item, or the item will be marked wrong.

Miscellaneous Testing Concerns

- Some states administer oral examinations. Some states administer examinations in languages other than English. These special examinations must be requested from your state testing agency when you register to take the test. If you think you need an oral examination or non-English version of the test, contact your instructor or state testing service for information and instructions.

- Your state will accommodate individuals with certain disabilities during the test. Contact your state testing agency in advance for information on requesting accommodations.

- Your state will have a skills (manual competency) examination portion of the state certification test. You must pass both portions of the test before being entered into the nurse aide registry. Contact your instructor or state testing agency for information.

- Do not bring children or visitors to the test site. These individuals will not be admitted.

- Do not bring pagers, telephones, or electronic devices to the test site. Use of these items will not be permitted.

Test Security

- Do not give help to or receive help from anyone during the test. If this occurs, the test will be stopped and your test will not be scored. You may be reported to your state nurse aide registry for this activity.

- Individuals caught removing a test from the testing site may be prosecuted.

Activities of Daily Living: Hygiene

1. Providing personal hygiene care:

a. is not very important to the elderly.

b. involves feeding and providing fluids.

c. may cause the client to feel ashamed.

d. does not require privacy.

Answer ➡

Activities of Daily Living: Hygiene

3. Oral hygiene involves:

a. cleaning the mouth, teeth, gums, and tongue.

b. rinsing the mouth with very cold water.

c. cleaning the mouth once a week.

d. scrubbing the tongue well with a toothbrush.

Answer ➡

Activities of Daily Living: Hygiene

2. When providing oral hygiene to a client with dentures:

a. brush the dentures with a toothbrush in the client's mouth.

b. remove the dentures and brush them using cool water.

c. scrub the dentures with mouthwash and very hot water.

d. soak the dentures in ice water to avoid damaging them with a brush.

Answer ➡

Activities of Daily Living: Hygiene

4. When assisting the client with perineal (peri) care:

a. begin wiping in the dirtiest area, working to the cleanest area.

b. scrub the perineum back and forth vigorously.

c. use plenty of soap and cool water to prevent skin irritation.

d. begin wiping in the cleanest area, working to the dirtiest area.

Answer ➡

ANSWER: b

Rationale:
The dentures are removed from the mouth and brushed to remove food particles. Cool water is used to avoid damaging the dentures.

ANSWER: d

Rationale:
Begin wiping in the cleanest area (near the urethra), working to the dirtiest area (the rectum) to avoid causing urinary and vaginal infections with the germs from the rectal area.

ANSWER: c

Rationale:
The client's body is exposed during personal hygiene care. He or she may be embarrassed because the body is exposed. The client may feel ashamed because she cannot care for herself.

ANSWER: a

Rationale:
Oral hygiene is done to clean the mouth, teeth, gums, and tongue. Food particles are removed. Regular oral hygiene promotes good health and makes the mouth feel fresh and clean. Good oral hygiene improves client self-confidence and self-esteem.

Activities of Daily Living: Hygiene

5. **You are assigned to give a client a partial bath during H.S. care. You will:**

a. give the client a bed bath.

b. wash the face, hands, underarms, and perineum.

c. give a tub bath to relax the client.

d. wash the hands and put the client to bed.

Answer ➡

Activities of Daily Living: Hygiene

6. **ADLs are:**

a. things clients buy at the store.

b. recreational activities.

c. social skills.

d. personal care activities.

Answer ➡

Activities of Daily Living: Hygiene

7. **A client's personal hygiene routines may be influenced by:**

a. the nurse aide's routine.

b. a family member's preferences.

c. culture.

d. the state survey agency rules.

Answer ➡

Activities of Daily Living: Hygiene

8. **When giving a complete bed bath, the nurse aide washes the:**

a. client's entire body.

b. hands, face, underarms, and perineum.

c. face, legs, perineum, and back.

d. face, hands, perineum, and feet.

Answer ➡

ANSWER: d

Rationale:
ADLs are activities of daily living. These are personal care activities that people do each day to meet their basic human needs. Personal hygiene is an ADL skill.

ANSWER: a

Rationale:
A complete bed bath (CBB) is given to dependent clients who must remain in bed. The client's entire body is bathed by the nurse aide.

ANSWER: b

Rationale:
H.S. care is given at bedtime. This abbreviation stands for "hour of sleep." A partial bath is commonly given for comfort and personal cleanliness. A partial bath involves washing the face, hands, underarms, and perineal area.

ANSWER: c

Rationale:
Hygiene is a very personal activity. Practices are often determined by the client's culture. The nurse aide should also consider client preferences for time of day and other requests.

Activities of Daily Living: Hygiene

10. **The purpose of assisting clients with daily hygienic care is to:**

a. prevent odors in the facility.

b. ensure that clients are clean and dry.

c. prevent pressure ulcers and contractures from developing.

d. prevent infection, promote relaxation, enhance self-esteem.

Answer ➥

Activities of Daily Living: Hygiene

12. **When you are preparing to give a client a bath, the room should be:**

a. warm and comfortable.

b. hot and humid.

c. cool and dry.

d. hot and dry.

Answer ➥

Activities of Daily Living: Hygiene

9. **When washing the client's face:**

a. use plenty of soap and hot water.

b. avoid the use of soap near the eyes.

c. ask the client if she prefers cool water.

d. begin with the neck and wash upward.

Answer ➥

Activities of Daily Living: Hygiene

11. **The temperature of the client's bath water should be approximately:**

a. 75 degrees.

b. 85 degrees.

c. 105 degrees.

d. 125 degrees.

Answer ➥

ANSWER: d

Rationale:
The benefits of daily hygiene are too numerous to list. Good hygiene is necessary for good health. Daily bathing and hygiene stimulate circulation, promote relaxation, reduce the risk of infection, eliminate odors, and enhance self-esteem.

ANSWER: a

Rationale:
The room temperature should be warm and comfortable to prevent chilling.

ANSWER: b

Rationale:
When washing the face, begin with the eye area. Avoid using soap near the eyes. Remember that the eyes are a mucous membrane; avoid touching mucous membranes with your ungloved hands. After you have washed the eyes, rinse the washcloth, then wash the rest of the face.

ANSWER: c

Rationale:
Bath water temperature should be approximately 105 degrees. Temperatures lower than this will be too cool and higher than this may cause burns.

Activities of Daily Living: Hygiene

13. The *primary* purpose of oral hygiene is to:

   a. remove medication residue and bad tastes caused by illness.

   b. clean the mouth, teeth, gums, and tongue.

   c. eliminate all bacteria from the mouth and teeth.

   d. prevent the spread of viral infection.

Answer ➥

Activities of Daily Living: Hygiene

14. Brush the client's teeth using:

   a. a very stiff brush.

   b. an up-and-down motion.

   c. a glycerin swab.

   d. a side-to-side motion.

Answer ➥

Activities of Daily Living: Hygiene

15. Store the client's dentures:

   a. wrapped in a paper towel in the drawer.

   b. in an emesis basin.

   c. in very hot water with a denture tablet.

   d. in a covered, labeled cup of cool water.

Answer ➥

Activities of Daily Living: Hygiene

16. The *primary* purpose of providing skin care is to:

   a. prevent complications, including infection and pressure ulcers.

   b. eliminate odors from the facility.

   c. remove urine and feces.

   d. make the client look attractive.

Answer ➥

ANSWER: b

Rationale:
Always brush the client's teeth using an up-and-down motion. This is most effective for removing trapped food particles from between the teeth and gums.

ANSWER: a

Rationale:
To some degree, all of the answers listed apply to skin care. However, "a" encompasses all of them. The primary purpose is to prevent infection and pressure ulcers. Proper skin care enhances circulation and promotes self-esteem.

ANSWER: b

Rationale:
The purpose of oral hygiene is to clean the mouth, teeth, gums, and tongue. This reduces bacteria and promotes good health. The client is more self-confident if his or her mouth and teeth are clean.

ANSWER: d

Rationale:
Dentures are stored in a covered cup that is labeled with the client's name. Use cool water to avoid damaging the dentures.

Activities of Daily Living: Hygiene

17. **When applying lotion to the client's back, the nurse aide should:**

    a. rub in small circles.

    b. massage red areas well to stimulate circulation.

    c. apply plenty of lotion and powder.

    d. rub the back and buttocks using firm, even strokes.

Answer ➧

Notes

Notes

Notes

Notes

ANSWER: d

Rationale:
Avoid massaging red or open areas. Rubbing in firm, even strokes is best. Massage the entire back and buttocks. Avoid a large amount of lotion, which may not be absorbed completely. Avoid powder, as the friction may cause skin irritation.

Activities of Daily Living: Dressing and Grooming

1. **When shaving a male client:**

   a. holding the skin taut, begin with the neck area.

   b. use long, upward strokes, beginning with the cheeks.

   c. rinse the razor after every 5 strokes.

   d. ask the client to tighten the upper lip when shaving.

Answer ☛

Activities of Daily Living: Dressing and Grooming

3. **Mrs. Huynh has an order for support (antiembolism) hosiery. You should:**

   a. ask the nurse to apply the hosiery.

   b. seat the client in a chair before applying the hosiery.

   c. apply the hose before Mrs. Huynh gets out of bed.

   d. place the hose over the toes and ask the client to pull them up.

Answer ☛

Activities of Daily Living: Dressing and Grooming

2. **When providing foot care to a diabetic client:**

   a. dry the feet and area between the toes well.

   b. clip the toenails very short to prevent injury.

   c. clean under the toenails with a nail file.

   d. apply lotion between the toes.

Answer ☛

Activities of Daily Living: Dressing and Grooming

4. **When dressing Mr. Keene, a 77-year-old client who has had a stroke, the nurse aide should:**

   a. apply the pants first.

   b. put the shirt on the affected arm first.

   c. put the pants on the unaffected leg first.

   d. position the client supine for dressing.

Answer ☛

ANSWER: a

Rationale:
Always avoid using sharp objects when caring for the feet of a client with diabetes. Do not cut the toenails of a client with diabetes. This is a licensed nursing responsibility. Avoid lotion between the toes, as this increases the risk of infection. Dry well between the toes, because bacteria grow best in a warm, moist, dark environment. Drying between the toes prevents infection, which can lead to serious complications in diabetics.

ANSWER: b

ANSWER: d

Rationale:
Begin shaving with the sideburns and cheeks, holding the skin taut and shaving in short, even strokes. Next, move to the upper lip. Ask the client to tighten the skin to avoid injury. Shave from the nose area to the upper lip in short, downward strokes.

ANSWER: c

Rationale:
Most clients are dressed while in the sitting position. When dressing a client with a paralyzed side from a stroke, always apply the clothes to the affected extremity first, followed by the unaffected side. Dressing the affected side first is easier, and reduces the risk of pain and injury to the client.

Rationale:
Apply the hose before the client gets out of bed. Once she is in the chair, her feet may swell, making the hose more difficult to apply. Antiembolism hose are difficult for clients to apply. This is a nurse aide responsibility.

Activities of Daily Living: Dressing and Grooming

6. **When undressing a client who has a paralyzed side from a stroke, the nurse aide should:**

   a. undress the affected (paralyzed) side first

   b. remove the pants first.

   c. undress the strong (unaffected) side first.

   d. have the client remove the shoes before beginning.

Answer ➥

Activities of Daily Living: Dressing and Grooming

8. **Mrs. Secrest has long hair that is tangled in the back. To remove the tangle, the nurse aide should:**

   a. hold the tangled section of the hair tight and begin combing at the end, working upward in short strokes.

   b. wet the hair thoroughly before attempting to remove the tangle.

   c. cut the tangled section carefully with scissors.

   d. wet only the tangled section of hair, then begin brushing it from the top, working downward in long, even strokes.

Answer ➥

Activities of Daily Living: Dressing and Grooming

5. **You are assigned to give Miss Kavalos a shower with shampoo. The client wears hearing aids in both ears. You should:**

   a. leave the hearing aids in her ears so she can hear your instructions.

   b. wash the hearing aids well when you shampoo the hair.

   c. dry the hearing aids thoroughly with a hair dryer after the shower.

   d. remove the hearing aids before showering the client.

Answer ➥

Activities of Daily Living: Dressing and Grooming

7. **A prosthesis is a/an:**

   a. ambulation aid.

   b. artificial body part.

   c. means of transportation.

   d. medical treatment.

Answer ➥

ANSWER: c

Rationale:
When undressing a client with weakness or paralysis, always remove the clothing from the strong side first. This will make removing the clothes from the affected side easier and reduce the risk of pain and injury to the client. In most cases, the client will be unable to remove the shoes. The nurse aide will have to remove them.

ANSWER: d

Rationale:
Always avoid getting hearing aids wet. Water will damage them. Remove them before showering the client. Store them in a safe location. Avoid exposing the hearing aids to sources of heat, such as a hair dryer, as this will also damage them.

ANSWER: a

Rationale:
Never cut a client's hair. Avoid pulling on the scalp when combing. To remove a tangle, begin by sectioning a small part of the hair with the comb. Hold the hair firmly above where you are combing. Begin at the bottom, working your way up to the area near the scalp. Use short, even, downward strokes.

ANSWER: b

Rationale:
A prosthesis is an artificial body part that is used when the client's body is no longer functioning or a part has been removed. Many prostheses are available, including artificial arms and legs and artificial eyes. The nurse aide must treat the prosthesis with respect, as part of the client's body.

Activities of Daily Living: Dressing and Grooming

10. The *primary* purpose of providing hand and nail care is to:

a. prevent clients from scratching staff during care.

b. prevent clients from scratching themselves.

c. promote good health and reduce the risk of infection.

d. ensure that clients wear nail polish if they want.

Answer ➡

Notes

Activities of Daily Living: Dressing and Grooming

9. When applying lotion to the client's skin, the nurse aide should:

a. avoid the face area.

b. rub the entire back and buttocks with gentle, firm strokes.

c. massage the legs well, using firm up-and-down strokes.

d. not apply lotion between the fingers, to prevent infection.

Answer ➡

Activities of Daily Living: Dressing and Grooming

11. When providing fingernail care to a client:

a. use a knife, paper clip, or file to remove dirt from under the nails.

b. use a paper clip or file to remove dirt from under the nails.

c. clip the nails back to the quick.

d. soak the hands in warm water and scrub under the nails with a soft brush.

Answer ➡

ANSWER: c

Rationale:
The primary purpose of hand and fingernail care is to cleanse the hands, to remove germs from the palms, fingers, and nail beds. Nail care also improves appearance and reduces the risk of injury from long or sharp nails.

NOTES

ANSWER: b

Rationale:
Many elderly clients have dry skin, so lotion may be used liberally. Never massage the legs. This action could dislodge a blood clot. If applying lotion to the legs, pat or rub it in gently. Avoid using lotion in the eyes, perineal area, and between the toes. Lotion may be used on all other areas, as the client prefers. When applying lotion to the back, use firm, gentle strokes. Massage the length of the back and buttocks area to stimulate circulation.

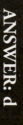

ANSWER: d

Rationale:
Avoid using sharp objects that may injure the client. Avoid clipping the nails too short, which may cause pain or injury. Soaking the hands in warm water is relaxing. Dirt under the nails is easily removed by scrubbing with a soft brush.

1. **Nutrients are:**
   a. unimportant byproducts of food.
   b. essential to life.
   c. chemical preservatives.
   d. liquids.

Answer ☞

2. **Carbohydrates:**
   a. prevent dehydration.
   b. are nature's building blocks.
   c. provide fuel and energy.
   d. should be limited.

Answer ☞

3. **Proteins:**
   a. are essential for good health, healing, and growth.
   b. provide empty calories and should be limited.
   c. are unimportant to most people.
   d. should be limited to six servings each day.

Answer ☞

4. **According to the Food Guide Pyramid, clients should consume:**
   a. 6 servings of dairy products each day.
   b. 4 to 6 servings of fat each day.
   c. 2 servings of bread, cereal, or pasta each day.
   d. 3 to 5 servings of vegetables each day.

Answer ☞

ANSWER: c

Rationale:
Carbohydrates are found in many foods, including grains, fruits, and vegetables. They are essential for good health and provide fuel and energy for the body.

ANSWER: b

Rationale:
Nutrients are essential to life. They include water, vitamins, minerals, carbohydrates, proteins, and fats.

ANSWER: d

Rationale:
According to the USDA Food Guide Pyramid, adults should consume 6-11 servings from the bread, rice, cereal, and pasta food group; 3-5 servings of vegetables; 2-4 servings of fruit; 2-3 servings of meat; and 2-3 servings of dairy products. Fats should be used sparingly.

ANSWER: a

Rationale:
Proteins are nature's building blocks and are essential for healing, growth, and overall good health. The meat, poultry, dry bean, egg, and nut food group provides the most protein.

Activities of Daily Living: Nutrition and Hydration

5. **Which of the following would be found on a clear liquid tray?**

   a. Tea with sugar.

   b. Pudding.

   c. Applesauce.

   d. Milk.

Answer ➣

Activities of Daily Living: Nutrition and Hydration

6. **Which of the following would be found on a full liquid tray?**

   a. Creamed spinach.

   b. Pears.

   c. Milkshake.

   d. Ground meat.

Answer ➣

Activities of Daily Living: Nutrition and Hydration

7. **A diabetic diet would *not* contain which of the following food items?**

   a. Salt.

   b. Pepper.

   c. Vinegar.

   d. Sugar.

Answer ➣

Activities of Daily Living: Nutrition and Hydration

8. **A nasogastric tube is:**

   a. inserted through the abdominal wall into the stomach.

   b. threaded through the nose into the stomach.

   c. used to drain urine from the bladder.

   d. used only for medication administration.

Answer ➣

ANSWER: c

Rationale:
The full liquid diet contains liquid food items. Many of these are milk-based. Of those listed, a milkshake is the only item that qualifies. The other foods listed are solids and are not included in a full liquid diet.

ANSWER: b

Rationale:
A nasogastric tube is used for feeding and medication administration. It is inserted into the nose and threaded into the stomach.

ANSWER: a

Rationale:
The clear liquid diet contains food items you can see through. Keeping this in mind, the only item listed above that qualifies is tea with sugar.

ANSWER: d

Rationale:
Clients with diabetes can have all of the food items listed here except sugar. If sweetener is needed, an artificial sugar substitute is used.

Activities of Daily Living:
Nutrition and Hydration

10. **When a client is being fed by tube, the nurse aide must always:**

    a. position the client in the lateral position.

    b. keep the bed flat.

    c. raise the side rails when the client is in bed.

    d. elevate the head of the bed.

Answer ➜

Activities of Daily Living:
Nutrition and Hydration

12. **Which of the following *would not* be included when recording intake and output?**

    a. Tea.

    b. Popsicles.

    c. Sherbet.

    d. Applesauce.

Answer ➜

Activities of Daily Living:
Nutrition and Hydration

9. **A gastrostomy tube is:**

    a. inserted through the abdominal wall into the stomach.

    b. threaded through the nose into the stomach.

    c. used to drain urine from the bladder.

    d. used only for medication administration.

Activities of Daily Living:
Nutrition and Hydration

11. **An order to force fluids involves:**

    a. forcing the client to drink a glass of water every hour.

    b. encouraging the client to drink each time you are in the room.

    c. giving liquids through a nasogastric tube.

    d. making the client drink only the liquids on the meal tray.

Answer ➜

ANSWER: d

Rationale:
The client's head must be elevated at all times during tube feeding and for 30 to 60 minutes after the feeding is finished, to prevent choking and aspiration.

ANSWER: a

Rationale:
A gastrostomy tube is used for feeding and medication administration. It is surgically inserted. The tube is inserted through the abdominal wall into the stomach.

ANSWER: d

Rationale:
When recording intake and output, record liquids or food items that become liquid at room temperature. Of the items listed, all are liquids or will melt to room temperature except applesauce, which is a blended food item.

ANSWER: b

Rationale:
We do not really force clients to drink liquids. An order to "force fluids" means to encourage the client to drink at every opportunity, including each time you are in the room. The objective is to encourage as much liquid intake as possible during your shift.

Activities of Daily Living: Nutrition and Hydration

13. When passing meal trays:

a. check the tray cards to ensure that you have the correct client and correct food on the tray.

b. pass all the feeder trays first by placing them on the client's table, then returning to spoon-feed after all trays are passed.

c. remove the covers from food items and leave them on the tray cart.

d. pass trays first, then return to assist clients in preparing and cutting the food.

Answer ➜

Activities of Daily Living: Nutrition and Hydration

14. When feeding clients:

a. serve all liquids last.

b. feed all hot foods first.

c. alternate liquids and solids.

d. withhold dessert if the client does not eat all of the other foods.

Answer ➜

Activities of Daily Living: Nutrition and Hydration

15. Food passes through the esophagus into the stomach, where:

a. it is eliminated quickly from the body.

b. it mixes with digestive enzymes before moving to the small intestine.

c. nutrients are absorbed for use by all body systems.

d. water and other liquids are absorbed for use by the kidneys.

Answer ➜

Activities of Daily Living: Nutrition and Hydration

16. Clients should consume enough fluid each day to:

a. prevent dehydration.

b. urinate every two hours.

c. balance their intake and output.

d. swallow their medications.

Answer ➜

ANSWER: c

Rationale: Feed slowly to prevent choking. Fill the spoon half full. Alternate liquids and solids. Never withhold food items from the client.

ANSWER: a

Rationale:
Always check the tray cards to ensure that you have the correct client and correct food items on the tray. Leave trays on the cart until you are ready to serve them. Leave food covered during transportation. Leave food covered during transportation. Do not place trays in front of clients until you are ready to feed them. Prepare the tray as needed at the time it is served so clients can begin eating immediately.

ANSWER: a

Rationale:
Adequate fluid is needed to prevent dehydration, a serious condition in the elderly. In most adults, 2 to 3 quarts of fluid are needed each day.

ANSWER: b

Rationale:
Food in the stomach mixes with digestive enzymes before moving into the small intestine.

Activities of Daily Living: Nutrition and Hydration

17. **Signs and symptoms of dehydration include:**

a. voiding frequently in small amounts.

b. lethargy, weakness, low blood pressure.

c. high fever, elevated blood pressure, dark circles under the eyes.

d. slow pulse, cyanosis, edema.

Answer ➜

ANSWER: b

Rationale:
Signs and symptoms of dehydration include lethargy, weakness, low blood pressure, rapid pulse, dry mucous membranes, sunken eyeballs, and tenting of the skin.

Activities of Daily Living: Elimination

1. Incontinence is:

a. a medical problem.

b. a normal part of aging.

c. normal for confused clients.

d. always a sign of infection.

Answer →

Activities of Daily Living: Elimination

2. Feces are:

a. liquid waste products.

b. bowel movements.

c. emesis.

d. perspiration.

Answer →

Activities of Daily Living: Elimination

3. Voiding is:

a. fecal elimination.

b. vomiting.

c. urination.

d. surgical drainage.

Answer →

Activities of Daily Living: Elimination

4. Fecal impaction is:

a. retaining fluids because of a kidney problem.

b. passage of liquid stool.

c. caused by indigestion.

d. the most serious form of constipation.

Answer →

ANSWER: b

Rationale:
The terms bowel movement, feces, and stool may be used interchangeably. These are solid waste products of the digestive process.

ANSWER: a

Rationale:
Incontinence is a medical problem that can often be corrected or improved. It is not a normal part of aging or mental confusion. It can be a sign of infection, but incontinence does not always indicate that infection is present. Clients should be taken to the bathroom as often as necessary to prevent incontinence.

ANSWER: d

Rationale: Fecal impaction is the most serious form of constipation. Bowel movements must be monitored to prevent constipation. If detected, fecal impaction must be relieved promptly. Passing liquid stool may be a sign of fecal impaction.

ANSWER: c

Rationale:
Voiding is the same as urination. This process involves eliminating liquid waste from the body.

Activities of Daily Living: Elimination

6. **When assisting a client to use the bedpan, position the bed in the:**

   a. Fowler's position.

   b. supine position.

   c. prone position.

   d. lateral position.

Answer ➔

Activities of Daily Living: Elimination

8. **When caring for a client with an indwelling catheter:**

   a. always position the drainage bag on the floor.

   b. position the drainage bag above the level of the bladder.

   c. position the drainage bag below the level of the bladder.

   d. always disconnect the catheter during bathing.

Answer ➔

Activities of Daily Living: Elimination

5. **A urinal is:**

   a. for elimination of solid waste products.

   b. used by male clients for urination.

   c. needed for care of female clients.

   d. the same as an emesis basin.

Answer ➔

Activities of Daily Living: Elimination

7. **The bedside commode is used for:**

   a. vomiting.

   b. males only.

   c. female clients.

   d. urinary and fecal elimination.

Answer ➔

ANSWER: a

Rationale:
Position the bed in the high Fowler's position, if possible. The Fowler's position is a semi-sitting position. The client must be seated upright for proper elimination.

ANSWER: b

Rationale: Male clients may use the urinal for passage of urine, a liquid waste product.

ANSWER: c

Rationale:
The urinary drainage bag must always be maintained below the level of the bladder. Avoid raising the bag above the bladder, which will cause urine to flow back into the bladder, increasing the risk of infection. Avoid placing the bag on the floor, which also increases the risk of infection.

ANSWER: d

Rationale:
The bedside commode is used for both male and female clients in place of a toilet. It may be used for both urinary and fecal elimination.

Activities of Daily Living: Elimination

9. The urinary catheter:

a. is always attached to the side rail when the client is in bed.

b. must be fastened to the client's leg or abdomen at all times.

c. is not fastened to the client's body when in bed.

d. is disconnected every shift so the tubing can be rinsed.

Answer ➔

Activities of Daily Living: Elimination

10. The organ in which urine is stored before leaving the body is the:

a. bladder.

b. ureter.

c. kidney.

d. urethra.

Answer ➔

Activities of Daily Living: Elimination

11. Water is absorbed from solid food waste in the:

a. stomach.

b. small intestine.

c. pancreas.

d. large intestine.

Answer ➔

Notes

ANSWER: a

Rationale:
The bladder is a hollow muscle that expands and contracts. Urine passes into the bladder from the kidneys. Urine remains in the bladder until it is eliminated from the body.

ANSWER: b

Rationale:
The catheter must be fastened to the client's leg (or abdomen in males) at all times. This prevents pulling on the catheter, which would cause it to dislodge. It also prevents discomfort and traction on the urethra.

ANSWER: d

Rationale:
Water is absorbed from stool in the large intestine. The digestive system slows in the elderly. If stool remains in the large intestine for a prolonged period, the risk of constipation and fecal impaction is increased.

Activities of Daily Living: Rest/Comfort/Sleep

1. Pain:

a. is normal in the elderly.

b. means something is wrong.

c. does not affect client behavior.

d. need not be reported.

Answer ➥

Activities of Daily Living: Rest/Comfort/Sleep

2. A confused client moans and makes a face when you reposition him in bed. This may be a sign of:

a. anger.

b. hunger.

c. thirst.

d. pain.

Answer ➥

Activities of Daily Living: Rest/Comfort/Sleep

3. A client who had her leg amputated two years ago complains of pain in her foot. You know that:

a. the pain is imaginary.

b. she wants attention.

c. the pain is normal.

d. she is having phantom pain.

Answer ➥

Activities of Daily Living: Rest/Comfort/Sleep

4. Comfort is a:

a. state of well-being.

b. state of confusion.

c. painful condition.

d. cause of restlessness.

Answer ➥

ANSWER: d

Rationale:
Moaning and grimacing are often signs of pain. Your observations should be reported promptly to the nurse in charge.

ANSWER: a

Rationale:
Comfort is a state of well-being. A client is in a state of comfort when he or she is not in pain or upset. He or she feels calm and relaxed. Many factors affect clients' comfort. Environmental factors include noise, odor, temperature, lighting, and ventilation.

ANSWER: b

Rationale:
Pain is never normal. The elderly suffer from many acute and chronic diseases that may cause pain. Pain is a warning that something is wrong. It should always be promptly reported to the nurse. Pain may cause clients to display behavior problems. Nursing comfort measures such as a warm bath, repositioning, or a backrub may be used to eliminate or reduce pain.

ANSWER: d

Rationale:
The client is having phantom pain. This pain is real, not imaginary. Phantom pain sometimes occurs after body parts have been removed.

Activities of Daily Living: Rest/Comfort/Sleep

6. **Assisting the client to relax may:**

   a. make the client more alert.

   b. cure physical problems.

   c. relieve anxiety, pain, and fear.

   d. reduce the desire to eat so much.

Answer ➔

Activities of Daily Living: Rest/Comfort/Sleep

8. **The need for sleep:**

   a. decreases with age.

   b. occurs on a fixed schedule in the elderly.

   c. increases with age.

   d. is not important to the elderly.

Answer ➔

Activities of Daily Living: Rest/Comfort/Sleep

5. **Comfort, rest, and sleep are necessary to:**

   a. escape from life's problems.

   b. relieve pain.

   c. restore strength and repair body problems.

   d. cure chronic diseases.

Answer ➔

Activities of Daily Living: Rest/Comfort/Sleep

7. **Before a client can rest comfortably, the nurse aide must:**

   a. turn off all the lights.

   b. ensure that hunger, thirst, and elimination needs are met.

   c. give the client a blanket.

   d. ask the nurse to give the client a sleeping pill.

Answer ➔

ANSWER: c

Rationale:
Relaxation has many helpful effects. Of those listed, the only one that has been scientifically proven is reduction of pain, anxiety, and fear.

ANSWER: a

Rationale:
The elderly generally need less sleep than younger persons.

ANSWER: c

Rationale:
Comfort, rest, and sleep are needed by all individuals to restore strength and energy, enabling the body to repair itself.

ANSWER: b

Rationale:
The client's basic needs must be met before he or she can rest comfortably. The client will be unable to rest if he is hungry, thirsty, in pain, or needs to use the bathroom.

Activities of Daily Living: Rest/Comfort/Sleep

9. **The purpose of sleep is to:**

   a. allow the client to escape from reality.

   b. provide rest and repair for the mind and body.

   c. eliminate the cares of life.

   d. relieve physical and emotional pain.

Answer ➤

Notes

Activities of Daily Living: Rest/Comfort/Sleep

10. **When positioning the client on the side in bed, support him or her:**

    a. with restraints.

    b. by using the side rails.

    c. with pillows.

    d. by elevating the head and knee rests.

Answer ➤

Notes

ANSWER: c

Rationale:
Placing pillows behind the back will support the client comfortably. The other methods listed here are not recommended except in certain circumstances.

NOTES

ANSWER: b

Rationale:
All mammals need sleep to rest and repair the mind and body. Adequate sleep is necessary for the body and mind to function properly.

NOTES

Basic Nursing Skills: Infection Control

1. Microbes that cause disease are:

   a. pathogens.

   b. vectors.

   c. fomites.

   d. hosts.

Answer ➔

Basic Nursing Skills: Infection Control

2. A person who can transmit an infection to others is a:

   a. vector.

   b. microorganism.

   c. carrier.

   d. reservoir.

Answer ➔

Basic Nursing Skills: Infection Control

3. You remove a client's clothes to give her a shower. A dressing falls from her hip onto the floor, revealing a minor wound. The wound is not bleeding, but there is a small amount of old, dried blood on the dressing. You should:

   a. pick the dressing up and put it in the open trash can.

   b. apply gloves and place the dressing in a plastic bag.

   c. get the nurse in charge at once.

   d. do nothing, as this is not a nurse aide responsibility.

Answer ➔

Basic Nursing Skills: Infection Control

4. You are instructed to collect a regular urine specimen from a female client. You should:

   a. collect the specimen from the bedpan.

   b. apply the principles of standard precautions when obtaining the specimen.

   c. collect feces the next time the client eliminates.

   d. apply gloves and hold the cup securely against the client's perineum.

Answer ➔

ANSWER: c

Rationale:
A carrier can transmit an infection to others. The carrier may not know that he or she is infected.

ANSWER: a

Rationale:
Pathogens are microbes that are always capable of causing disease or infection. Vectors and fomites are vehicles that can transmit disease. The host is a place where pathogens can grow.

ANSWER: b

Rationale:
Always apply the principles of standard precautions when handling laboratory specimens. This will protect both the nurse aide and the client.

ANSWER: b

Rationale:
The dressing is contaminated with blood, so do not touch it with your bare hands. Avoid placing it in an open container. The dressing should be discarded in the biohazardous waste. Do not leave the client alone to get the nurse. The wound is minor and is not bleeding, so getting the nurse immediately is not critical. Use the call signal to notify the nurse.

Basic Nursing Skills:
Infection Control

6. **An example of the direct contact mode of transmission of infection is:**

   a. touching an infected wound.

   b. sneezing.

   c. coughing.

   d. contacting soiled bed linens.

Answer ➤

Basic Nursing Skills:
Infection Control

8. **Standard precautions are used:**

   a. only when clients have an infection.

   b. routinely in the care of all clients.

   c. only when giving perineal care.

   d. when it is part of your assignment.

Answer ➤

Basic Nursing Skills:
Infection Control

5. **You are assigned to collect a midstream urine specimen from a male client. You must:**

   a. apply gloves and collect the specimen in a clean cup.

   b. use a condom catheter to collect the specimen properly.

   c. pour the specimen from a urinal into the specimen cup.

   d. wash the perineum first to prevent specimen contamination.

Answer ➤

Basic Nursing Skills:
Infection Control

7. **The best method of preventing the spread of infection is:**

   a. wearing gloves.

   b. isolating clients with known infection.

   c. frequent handwashing.

   d. keeping clean and dirty items separate.

Answer ➤

ANSWER: a

Rationale:
Touching an infected wound is an example of direct contact. Sneezing and coughing are methods of airborne transmission. Contacting soiled linen is a method of direct contact transmission.

ANSWER: b

Rationale:
Standard precautions are used for all clients. Clients can be infectious without having obvious signs of infection. Standard precautions are used for all blood, body fluids (except sweat), secretions, excretions, mucous membranes, and nonintact skin.

ANSWER: d

Rationale:
A midstream specimen is always collected in a sterile container. The penis is washed to avoid specimen contamination. The client begins to void into the urinal or toilet. He must stop the urine stream, then void in the specimen cup. Avoid touching the inside of the cup with your fingers.

ANSWER: c

Rationale:
Frequent handwashing has been scientifically proven to be the best method of preventing the spread of infection. The other methods listed here are also important.

Basic Nursing Skills: Infection Control

10. **The nurse aide should wash his or her hands:**

a. after client care only.

b. before and after caring for each client.

c. only at the beginning and end of the shift.

d. once or twice a day.

Answer ➥

Basic Nursing Skills: Infection Control

12. **In addition to handwashing and wearing gloves, the use of standard precautions involves:**

a. wearing a mask when clients are in contact precautions.

b. understanding how pathogens are spread and using barrier equipment to protect yourself.

c. wearing full protective apparel when clients are in airborne and droplet precautions.

d. using paper dishes to serve meals to clients who are in isolation.

Answer ➥

Basic Nursing Skills: Infection Control

9. **Hepatitis B is transmitted through:**

a. the airborne method of transmission.

b. contact with inanimate objects.

c. improper handwashing techniques.

d. blood and body fluid transmission.

Answer ➥

Basic Nursing Skills: Infection Control

11. **The use of medical asepsis is important to:**

a. prevent the spread of infection.

b. maintain an attractive appearance.

c. make a good impression on others.

d. promote self-esteem.

Answer ➥

ANSWER: b

Rationale:
Frequent handwashing is important. The nurse aide should perform the handwashing procedure many times throughout the day. Of the choices listed here, always wash hands before and after caring for each client.

ANSWER: d

Rationale:
Hepatitis B is a bloodborne pathogen that is transmitted through blood and body fluid contact.

ANSWER: b

Rationale:
To use standard precautions properly, the nurse aide must understand the various methods by which infections are spread. The nurse aide will apply personal protective equipment (barrier equipment) to protect himself or herself.

ANSWER: a

Rationale:
Medical asepsis is an important part of the nurse aide's routine. Using medical asepsis correctly prevents the spread of infection.

Basic Nursing Skills:
Infection Control

14. The nurse aide is responsible for cleaning client care supplies and equipment to:

a. make the facility look neat and clean.

b. reduce odors.

c. make a good impression on others.

d. prevent the spread of infection.

Answer ➠

Basic Nursing Skills:
Infection Control

16. After client care items have been cleaned and disinfected, they should be stored in the:

a. clean utility room.

b. soiled utility room.

c. janitor closet.

d. linen room.

Answer ➠

Basic Nursing Skills:
Infection Control

13. Waste products that are contaminated with blood or body fluids:

a. are discarded in the open trash can in the client's room.

b. may be safely placed next to clean items.

c. are discarded in leakproof, covered containers.

d. do not require any special handling.

Answer ➠

Basic Nursing Skills:
Infection Control

15. When cleaning soiled client care items, the nurse aide should:

a. ask the charge nurse for advice.

b. wear personal protective equipment.

c. work in the clean utility room.

d. wrap all items as soon as they are washed.

Answer ➠

ANSWER: d

Rationale:
Some client care items must be cleaned regularly to prevent the spread of infection to clients, nurse aides, other staff, visitors, and others.

ANSWER: c

Rationale:
Waste materials contaminated with blood and body fluids are considered biohazardous and require special handling. These items are discarded in covered, leakproof containers.

ANSWER: a

Rationale:
Clean items are stored in the clean utility room. Soiled items are washed in the soiled utility room.

ANSWER: b

Rationale:
Based on knowledge of the way infection is spread, the nurse aide must select the correct personal protective equipment to use during cleaning procedures.

Basic Nursing Skills:
Infection Control

17. **When positioning supplies in the client's room, the nurse aide should:**

a. place the bedpan on the overbed table so the client can reach it.

b. keep the urinal in the bedside stand next to the washbasin.

c. keep clean and dirty items separate in the bedside stand.

d. store extra clean linens in the bedside stand so they are readily available.

Answer ➡

Basic Nursing Skills:
Infection Control

18. **Head lice:**

a. hop and fly from one person to another.

b. are spread by shared combs, brushes, and bedding.

c. are not easily spread.

d. are not a problem in the elderly.

Answer ➡

Basic Nursing Skills:
Infection Control

19. **Signs and symptoms of scabies include:**

a. a burning sensation.

b. tiny bugs crawling on the skin and bedding.

c. nits.

d. rash and intense itching.

Answer ➡

Basic Nursing Skills:
Infection Control

20. **A client who is newly diagnosed with head lice or scabies:**

a. is isolated in contact precautions

b. is isolated in airborne precautions.

c. is isolated in droplet precautions.

d. requires no special isolation measures.

Answer ➡

ANSWER: b

Rationale:
Head lice are spread on shared personal care items, and by direct contact. They do not hop or fly, but they can crawl very fast.

ANSWER: c

Rationale:
Clean and dirty items must be kept separate. The overbed table is a clean area used for eating, so avoid placing the bedpan or urinal on it. Keep clean items separate from dirty items in the bedside stand.

ANSWER: a

Rationale:
A client who is newly diagnosed with head lice or scabies is isolated in contact precautions for at least 24 hours after treatment. The room must be cleaned and all belongings washed before the client is removed from isolation.

ANSWER: d

Rationale:
Scabies is caused by microscopic mites that cannot be seen by the human eye. They cause a rash that is common to certain areas of the body, but may be widespread. Scabies causes intense itching.

Basic Nursing Skills: Safety/Emergency

2. The nurse aide walks into a client's room. The client is smoking in the room and set his trash can on fire when emptying an ashtray. The first action to take is to:

a. get the nurse in charge.

b. run for the fire extinguisher.

c. remove the client from the room.

d. use the blanket to smother the fire.

Answer ➜

Basic Nursing Skills: Safety/Emergency

4. A client is using oxygen. You enter the room and notice that he has turned the flow meter up all the way. You should:

a. turn the unit down at once.

b. notify the nurse in charge.

c. tell the client to leave the unit alone.

d. pretend you didn't notice the change in flow rate.

Answer ➜

Basic Nursing Skills: Safety/Emergency

1. A client is eating lunch when you notice his hands at his throat. The first thing you should do is:

a. ask the client if he can speak.

b. perform the Heimlich maneuver.

c. slap the client sharply on the back.

d. quickly get the nurse in charge.

Answer ➜

Basic Nursing Skills: Safety/Emergency

3. You must use the fire extinguisher to put out a trash fire in the stairwell. You should:

a. aim the hose at the top of the flames so the water falls over the fire.

b. sweep the hose from side to side in a three-foot circle surrounding the fire.

c. aim the extinguisher before removing the pin from the handle.

d. aim the extinguisher at the base of the fire and spray from side to side.

Answer ➜

ANSWER: c

Rationale:
The first step in a fire emergency is to remove clients from the area. Close the door to the room to contain the fire, then activate the alarm.

ANSWER: a

Rationale:
Hands at the throat is the universal sign for choking. However, you can injure the client by performing procedures that are not necessary. Before taking any action, ask the client if he can speak. If so, he is moving enough air to breathe. If he cannot speak, his airway is obstructed. The next step is to perform the Heimlich maneuver. Do not leave the client alone. Send someone else for the nurse or use the call signal.

ANSWER: b

Rationale:
The nurse aide is not permitted to adjust the oxygen flow rate. Notify the nurse in charge.

ANSWER: d

Rationale:
Remember the PASS system when using a fire extinguisher. First, Pull the pin from the handle of the extinguisher. Then Aim the hose at the base of the fire. Squeeze the handle to discharge the contents. Sweep the extinguisher from side to side while keeping it aimed at the base of the fire.

Basic Nursing Skills:
Safety/Emergency

6. The charge nurse directs you to apply a cool compress to Mr. Long's right ankle. You know that:

a. the compress should be left in place for at least an hour.

b. the skin under the compress should be checked every 10 minutes.

c. the compress will cause the skin to become very red.

d. the compress should be left in place for no more than 5 minutes.

Answer ➔

Basic Nursing Skills:
Safety/Emergency

8. An emergency call signal is sounding in Room 108. The nurse aide assigned to that room is on her lunch break. You should:

a. notify the nurse in charge.

b. go to the break room to get the nurse aide who is assigned to Room 108.

c. answer the signal and ask the client how you can help.

d. ignore the signal, as this is not your responsibility.

Answer ➔

Basic Nursing Skills:
Safety/Emergency

5. A client has fallen to the floor. She complains of severe pain in her left thigh. The nurse aide should:

a. stay with the client and use the call signal to get help.

b. get the nurse in charge right away.

c. lift the client back to bed.

d. put a pillow under the client's left leg.

Answer ➔

Basic Nursing Skills:
Safety/Emergency

7. A bedfast client is vomiting. The nurse aide should:

a. get the nurse in charge immediately.

b. turn the client on her abdomen.

c. clean up the mess at once.

d. turn the client's head to the side.

Answer ➔

ANSWER: b

Rationale:
Redness under a compress may be a sign of tissue injury. Check the skin under the compress every 10 minutes. If abnormalities are noted, remove it and notify the nurse.

ANSWER: c

Rationale:
Nurse aides are responsible for caring for all clients on the unit. Answering call signals is everyone's responsibility.

ANSWER: a

Rationale:
Always stay with the client in an emergency and provide any appropriate emergency measures that you are trained and qualified to provide. Never move a client from the floor until after he or she has been checked by the nurse.

ANSWER: d

Rationale:
A client who is vomiting is at risk of aspiration. Turn the client's head or body to the side at once to prevent secretions from entering the airway.

Basic Nursing Skills: Safety/Emergency

10. **When entering and leaving the client's room, the nurse aide must:**

   a. check for and correct any safety hazards.

   b. make sure the bed is in the high position.

   c. raise the side rails to protect the client.

   d. leave the door open at all times.

Answer ➔

Basic Nursing Skills: Safety/Emergency

12. **Side rails:**

   a. must always be raised when the client is in bed.

   b. are used only when ordered by the physician or needed by the client.

   c. can be dangerous if clients try to get out of bed.

   d. increase the risk of falls and serious injury in some clients.

Answer ➔

Basic Nursing Skills: Safety/Emergency

9. **A client is bleeding heavily from an injury. The nurse aide should:**

   a. run and get the nurse in charge.

   b. apply a bandage to the injury.

   c. quickly wrap the area with a towel.

   d. apply pressure with a gloved hand.

Answer ➔

Basic Nursing Skills: Safety/Emergency

11. **You see a newspaper and a shoe in the middle of the floor of the client's room. You should:**

   a. leave these items alone, as they are the client's personal property.

   b. kick the newspaper and shoe under the bed so they are out of the way.

   c. pick them up and place them in the proper location.

   d. ignore them, as they are not your responsibility.

Answer ➔

ANSWER: a

Rationale:
The nurse aide must always be aware of client safety. Check for and correct unsafe conditions upon entering and before leaving the client's room.

ANSWER: b

Rationale:
Side rails are restraints that can cause serious injury in certain circumstances. They are used only with a physician order or when needed by the client for turning and transferring.

ANSWER: d

Rationale:
Applying firm hand pressure is the best method of stopping bleeding. However, you must practice standard precautions. To do this, always apply gloves before contacting blood.

ANSWER: c

Rationale:
Pick them up and ask the client where to put them. Do not kick the items under the bed. The client may fall if he or she tries to retrieve them. Maintaining safety in the client's room is an important nurse aide responsibility.

Basic Nursing Skills: Safety/Emergency

13. The fire and disaster evacuation plan:

a. does not apply to the nurse aide.

b. is important only to the fire department.

c. is posted on the wall and used in certain emergencies.

d. is kept in the administrator's office for safekeeping.

Answer ➜

Basic Nursing Skills: Safety/Emergency

15. The fire alarm sounds. The facility is filling with smoke, but you do not see any flames. You should:

a. move clients behind a fire door and close the door.

b. begin evacuating all clients to the outside of the building.

c. ask the nurse in charge for instructions.

d. notify the administrator.

Answer ➜

Basic Nursing Skills: Safety/Emergency

14. You must remove Mrs. Vasquez from her room during a fire emergency. The client cannot walk. She is sitting in a heavy recliner without wheels. No wheelchair is available. The best way to move the client is to:

a. pick her up and carry her.

b. run down the hallway to see if a wheelchair is available.

c. move the furniture and try to push the recliner.

d. place her on a sheet or blanket and drag her.

Answer ➜

Basic Nursing Skills: Safety/Emergency

16. Safety is:

a. the nurse aide's responsibility.

b. everyone's responsibility.

c. the administrator's responsibility.

d. the housekeeper's responsibility.

Answer ➜

ANSWER: d

Rationale:
Remember that this is an emergency, and time is critical. Do not waste time trying to move furniture. Do not leave the client to find a wheelchair. Likewise, if the recliner is heavy and does not have wheels, do not try to move it. The safest, fastest way is to place the client on a sheet or blanket on the floor and drag her to a safe area.

ANSWER: b

Rationale:
Safety is everyone's responsibility. Maintaining a safe environment in the health care facility is a team effort. This effort pays off in a safe working environment for staff members and a safe living environment for clients.

ANSWER: c

Rationale:
The fire and disaster evacuation plan is a chart that is posted on the wall in a prominent location. The nurse aide must be familiar with it in the event evacuation becomes necessary.

ANSWER: a

Rationale:
Smoke kills more people than flames in a fire. Move all clients behind a fire door and close the door to prevent the spread of smoke and flames.

Basic Nursing Skills: Safety/Emergency

17. **The elements necessary for a fire to start are:**

a. matches, rags, and chemicals.

b. heat, oxygen, and fuel.

c. cigarettes, trash, and old clothes.

d. papers, trash, and dirt.

Answer ➜

Basic Nursing Skills: Safety/Emergency

18. **The purpose of using good body mechanics is to:**

a. prevent injury to the nurse aide and client.

b. enable the nurse aide to lift a heavier load than normal.

c. eliminate the need for special lifting equipment.

d. eliminate the need for extra personnel to help with transfers.

Answer ➜

Basic Nursing Skills: Safety/Emergency

19. **When lifting a heavy client or object, the nurse aide should:**

a. bend from the waist, using the strong back muscles to do the job.

b. keep the feet close together and bend from the hips.

c. tighten the abdominal muscles and use the strong arm muscles for lifting.

d. maintain a wide base of support, keep the back straight, and use the leg muscles.

Answer ➜

Basic Nursing Skills: Safety/Emergency

20. **Mr. Mayo is a dependent client who is 6'2" and weighs 375 pounds. To transfer him from the bed to a chair, the nurse aide should:**

a. use a transfer belt.

b. ask another nurse aide to help.

c. use the mechanical lift and at least one more nurse aide.

d. ask 3 other nurse aides to help you lift the client.

Answer ➜

ANSWER: a

Rationale:
Good body mechanics involve using good posture and the largest, strongest muscles available to do the job. Using good body mechanics prevents injury to both the nurse aide and the client.

ANSWER: b

Rationale:
A fire cannot start unless three elements are present. These are heat (a source of ignition), oxygen, and fuel.

ANSWER: c

Rationale:
The client is dependent, so he will not be able to help much with the transfer. Because of his large size, lifting this client may cause injury to the client, the nurse aide, or both. Of the choices listed, the mechanical lift is the safest. However, never use the lift alone. One or more nurse aides should be involved with this transfer for the sake of every-one's safety.

ANSWER: d

Rationale:
The back muscles are small, weak, and prone to injury. When lifting a client or heavy object, keep your back straight. Keep your feet apart to maintain a wide base of support. Bend from the knees and use the strong thigh and leg muscles to lift the client or object.

Basic Nursing Skills: Safety/Emergency

21. **You are ambulating Mr. Chang in the hallway with a gait belt when he begins to fall. You should:**

a. grasp the belt firmly and hold Mr. Chang up until help arrives.

b. pull the belt toward your body and ease the client down your leg to the floor.

c. call for another nurse aide to bring a chair to seat the client in.

d. let go of the belt and allow Mr. Chang to slide down to the floor slowly.

Answer

Notes

Notes

Notes

Notes

ANSWER: b

Rationale:
If a client begins to fall, pull him close to your body. Maintain a wide base of support, keeping your back straight. Guide the client to the floor. Protect the head.

Basic Nursing Skills:
Therapeutic/Technical Procedures

1. When making an occupied bed, you should:

a. raise the side rail on the opposite side of the bed.

b. lower both side rails to make it easier to make the bed.

c. place the soiled linen on the floor when you remove it.

d. remove the top linen first.

Answer ➡

Basic Nursing Skills:
Therapeutic/Technical Procedures

3. At the beginning of your shift, you notice that a client's restraint is tied too tightly. The client is struggling to free herself from the restraint. You should:

a. get the nurse in charge at once.

b. loosen the restraint and tie it correctly.

c. cut the strap to remove the restraint quickly.

d. apply a different type of restraint.

Answer ➡

Basic Nursing Skills:
Therapeutic/Technical Procedures

2. When making the bed:

a. bring extra linen into the room in case it is needed.

b. carry the clean linen close to your body.

c. hold the soiled linen away from your uniform.

d. place the soiled linen on the overbed table

Answer ➡

Basic Nursing Skills:
Therapeutic/Technical Procedures

4. Restraints should be tied:

a. in a square knot.

b. to the side rails.

c. in a quick-release (slip) knot.

d. to the armrest of the chair.

Answer ➡

ANSWER: c

Rationale:
Always hold clean and soiled linen away from your uniform. The clean linen is fresh from the laundry but will become contaminated if it contacts your uniform. The soiled linen has been in contact with a client and will contaminate your uniform.

ANSWER: c

Rationale:
Restraints should be fastened in a quick-release or slip knot so that they can be removed quickly in the event of an emergency.

ANSWER: a

Rationale:
When making an occupied bed, raise the bed to a good working height for you. Raise the rail on the opposite side from where you are working to protect the client. When you are finished, return the bed to the lowest horizontal position.

ANSWER: b

Rationale:
There is no reason to cut the restraint if it is tied correctly. If the restraint shows signs of being too tight, release the ties and reapply it correctly. If the client is restless, consider ambulating her or taking her to the bathroom before reapplying the restraint.

Basic Nursing Skills: Therapeutic/Technical Procedures

6. **You are instructed to take an axillary temperature. You know that this is:**

   a. the most accurate method of taking the temperature.

   b. taken by placing the thermometer under the arm.

   c. taken by placing the thermometer in the mouth.

   d. taken by placing the thermometer in the rectum.

Answer ➔

Basic Nursing Skills: Therapeutic/Technical Procedures

8. **The systolic blood pressure reading is the:**

   a. pressure when the heart is working.

   b. pressure when the heart is resting.

   c. same as the pulse rate.

   d. pulse pressure plus 10.

Answer ➔

Basic Nursing Skills: Therapeutic/Technical Procedures

5. **Restraints must be released every:**

   a. 15 minutes.

   b. 30 minutes.

   c. hour for 5 minutes.

   d. 2 hours for 10 minutes.

Answer ➔

Basic Nursing Skills: Therapeutic/Technical Procedures

7. **Which of the following vital signs should be reported to the nurse?**

   a. 98-120-28, 114/66

   b. 97² (Ax)-88-18-128/84

   c. 994 (R)-76-20-106/70

   d. 988-96-16-130/88

Answer ➔

ANSWER: b

Rationale:
The axillary temperature is the least accurate method of taking a temperature. It is taken by placing the tip of the thermometer under the arm and holding it in place. The axillary temperature is recorded by charting an (Ax) after the reading.

ANSWER: a

Rationale:
The systolic pressure is the pressure when the heart is contracting, or working.

ANSWER: d

Rationale:
Restraints must be released every 2 hours for 10 minutes. During this time, the client should be repositioned, ambulated, exercised, and/or taken to the bathroom.

ANSWER: a

Rationale:
The pulse and respirations are elevated in "a." The other vital signs listed for this question are all within normal limits.

Basic Nursing Skills:
Therapeutic/Technical Procedures

10. **When making an unoccupied bed, the nurse aide should:**

    a. make one side of the bed before moving to the other side.

    b. shake the soiled linen to check for lost items before placing it in the hamper.

    c. work from the bottom of the bed to the top.

    d. raise the side rails when finished making the bed.

Answer ☛

Basic Nursing Skills:
Therapeutic/Technical Procedures

12. **When moving the client toward the head of the bed, the nurse aide should:**

    a. raise the head of the bed to the sitting position.

    b. lower the head of the bed before moving the client.

    c. pull the client up by grasping the underarm area firmly.

    d. elevate the client's head on two pillows.

Answer ☛

Basic Nursing Skills:
Therapeutic/Technical Procedures

9. **You are assigned to weigh Mrs. Long using the wheelchair scale. Her weight is 22 pounds less than it was last month. You should:**

    a. inform the nurse immediately.

    b. balance the scale and recheck the weight.

    c. fill out a maintenance slip to check the scale.

    d. record the weight on the flow sheet; no other action is necessary.

Answer ☛

Basic Nursing Skills:
Therapeutic/Technical Procedures

11. **Before transferring a client from a wheelchair to the bed, the nurse aide should:**

    a. raise the bed to the highest horizontal position.

    b. position the wheelchair against the wall.

    c. lock the brakes on the wheelchair.

    d. position the chair so the client moves toward the weak side.

Answer ☛

ANSWER: a

Rationale:
Make one side of the bed completely before moving to the other side. This method is faster and conserves your energy. Avoid shaking the linen, which spreads germs. Check the linen for lost items when you remove it. Place the bed in the lowest horizontal position, with the side rails down, when you are finished.

ANSWER: b

Rationale:
Lower the head of the bed and remove the pillow before moving the client.

ANSWER: b

Rationale:
A weight loss of 22 pounds is fairly large for a 30-day period of time. This could indicate a serious medical problem, but more than likely is caused by a problem with the scale. The best course of action is to check the balance on the scale and recheck the weight. If still abnormal, report the weight loss to the nurse.

ANSWER: c

Rationale:
For safety, always lock the brakes to the wheelchair when transferring the client. The wheels on the bed should also be locked.

Basic Nursing Skills:
Therapeutic/Technical Procedures

14. **The primary purpose of elevating the bed to the proper working height when making the bed is to:**

a. make the procedure go faster.

b. prevent injury to your back.

c. reassure the client.

d. make it easier to disinfect the mattress.

Answer ➔

Basic Nursing Skills:
Therapeutic/Technical Procedures

16. **When providing postmortem care, the nurse aide should:**

a. always remove the dentures and place them in the drawer.

b. always apply the principles of standard precautions.

c. leave the door to the room open.

d. position the body on the side.

Answer ➔

Basic Nursing Skills:
Therapeutic/Technical Procedures

13. **The best method for moving a dependent client up in bed is to:**

a. use a mechanical lifter.

b. get plenty of extra help.

c. use the logroll procedure.

d. use a lift sheet.

Answer ➔

Basic Nursing Skills:
Therapeutic/Technical Procedures

15. **When operating a manual hospital bed, raise the head by:**

a. operating the handle on the right side.

b. releasing the lever under the mattress.

c. turning the handle on the left side.

d. turning the handle at the center of the bed.

Answer ➔

ANSWER: b

Rationale:
The purpose of raising the high-low bed is to prevent injury to the nurse aide's back. However, you must lower the bed to the lowest horizontal position when you leave the bed-side.

ANSWER: d

Rationale:
Of the methods listed, a lift sheet is the easiest for the nurse aide and risks the least amount of trauma to the client. However, you must prevent the client's heels from dragging across the surface of the bottom sheet during the procedure.

ANSWER: b

Rationale:
The body can be infectious after death. Always apply the principles of standard precautions.

ANSWER: c

Rationale:
The gatch handle on the left side of the foot of the bed is always used to elevate the head of the bed. The center handle controls bed height. The handle on the right positions the knee rest.

Basic Nursing Skills:
Data Collection and Reporting

1. You are assigned to collect I&O on Mr. Gonsalves. For lunch, he consumed an 8-ounce glass of milk, 2 ounces of water, and 4 ounces of ice cream. How many cc (ml) of fluid did he consume?

a. 240 cc.

b. 420 cc.

c. 4200 cc.

d. 140 cc.

Answer ➙

Basic Nursing Skills:
Data Collection and Reporting

2. When collecting the urinary output measurement (I&O) from a client with a catheter, the nurse aide should:

a. measure the urine into a graduate pitcher.

b. measure the urine into a bedpan or urinal.

c. use the markings on the side of the catheter bag to measure the urine.

d. estimate the amount of urine in the bag and record this amount.

Answer ➙

Basic Nursing Skills:
Data Collection and Reporting

3. The nurse asks you to take a client's blood pressure stat. You know this means:

a. before the end of the shift.

b. with the client lying stationary.

c. within the hour.

d. immediately.

Answer ➙

Basic Nursing Skills:
Data Collection and Reporting

4. A client with cyanosis has:

a. flushed skin.

b. blue or blue/gray color.

c. edema.

d. normal skin.

Answer ➙

ANSWER: a

Rationale:
The markings on the side of the catheter bag are not accurate. The most accurate method of recording the output is to empty the catheter into a graduate, then read the amount in the container at eye level.

ANSWER: b

Rationale:
Mr. Gonsalves drank 14 ounces. There are 30 cc in an ounce. 14 x 30 = 420 cc.

ANSWER: b

Rationale:
Cyanosis is the medical term for blue. Cyanosis is a serious condition. Clients may appear blue or blue/gray in color. In persons of color, the lips, nail beds, or mucous membranes have a blue appearance.

ANSWER: d

Rationale:
A stat procedure must be performed immediately, without delay.

Basic Nursing Skills: Data Collection and Reporting

5. Q.I.D. means:

a. 4 times a day.

b. 3 times a day.

c. 2 times a day.

d. once daily.

Answer →

Basic Nursing Skills: Data Collection and Reporting

6. T.I.D. means:

a. 4 times a day.

b. 3 times a day.

c. 2 times a day.

d. once daily.

Answer →

Basic Nursing Skills: Data Collection and Reporting

7. Edema is the medical term used to report:

a. vomiting.

b. cyanosis.

c. swelling.

d. pain.

Answer →

Basic Nursing Skills: Data Collection and Reporting

8. Emesis is the medical term used to report:

a. pain.

b. aspiration.

c. swelling.

d. vomiting.

Answer →

ANSWER: b

Rationale:
T.I.D. is the abbreviation for 3 times a day.

ANSWER: d

Rationale:
Emesis is the medical term for vomiting.

ANSWER: a

Rationale:
Q.I.D. is the abbreviation for 4 times a day.

ANSWER: c

Rationale:
Edema is the medical term for swelling.

Basic Nursing Skills:
Data Collection and Reporting

9. Mrs. Kosmacek left 5% of her meat and 75% of her vegetable on her tray before announcing that she was full. She ate all the bread, fruit, and dessert. She drank all her milk. You will record her food consumption as:

a. 25%.

b. 60%.

c. 75%.

d. 100%.

Answer ➥

Basic Nursing Skills:
Data Collection and Reporting

11. Record 3:40 P.M. in military time.

a. 0340.

b. 1540.

c. 3400.

d. 1604.

Answer ➥

Basic Nursing Skills:
Data Collection and Reporting

10. Record 7:20 P.M. in military time.

a. 0720.

b. 2007.

c. 7200.

d. 1920.

Answer ➥

Basic Nursing Skills:
Data Collection and Reporting

12. You are assigned to measure the height of a bedfast client. You should:

a. use a ruler to measure from the top of the head to the feet.

b. measure from the top of the head to the tip of the toes with a yardstick.

c. inform the nurse that the client cannot be measured.

d. measure the height from head to heel using a tape measure.

Answer ➥

ANSWER: d

Rationale:
Using the 24-hour clock, 7:20 P.M. is recorded as 1920.

ANSWER: c

Rationale:
The intake is approximately 75% if the majority of the meal is consumed, but a significant amount of one or more food items is left over.

ANSWER: d

Rationale:
Use a tape measure to measure from the top of the client's head to the heel. An alternate method is to make a pencil mark on the sheet at the top of the head and another at the heels. Measure the distance between the two marks with a tape measure.

ANSWER: b

Rationale:
Using the 24-hour clock, 3:40 P.M. is recorded as 1540.

Basic Nursing Skills:
Data Collection and Reporting

13. **When weighing the client with a bed scale, the nurse aide should:**

a. cover the client with the bed linen so he or she does not get cold.

b. make sure the client swings freely in the sling from side to side.

c. subtract the weight of the sling from the total weight.

d. ensure that the sling hangs freely and the client's body does not touch the bed.

Answer ➡

Basic Nursing Skills:
Data Collection and Reporting

14. **Before weighing a client on a standing balance scale, the nurse aide should:**

a. balance the scale.

b. remove the client's clothing.

c. disinfect the scale.

d. raise the height bar.

Answer ➡

Basic Nursing Skills:
Data Collection and Reporting

15. **A client vomits a substance that looks like coffee grounds. The nurse aide should:**

a. clean it up and advise the nurse at the end of the shift.

b. notify the nurse immediately.

c. document the appearance of the emesis.

d. give the client an emesis basin.

Answer ➡

Basic Nursing Skills:
Data Collection and Reporting

16. **A client is voiding frequently in small amounts. Her urine is foul-smelling. The nurse aide should:**

a. apply an extra incontinent pad.

b. take the client to the bathroom every hour.

c. notify the nurse of these observations.

d. record the observations on an I&O sheet.

Answer ➡

ANSWER: a

Rationale:
The scale must be balanced (calibrated) to obtain an accurate weight. Always balance the scale before beginning the procedure.

ANSWER: d

Rationale:
For an accurate weight, the sling must be suspended off the surface of the bed. The client's body should not contact the surface of the bed when the weight is recorded.

ANSWER: c

Rationale:
The signs listed here suggest a urinary tract infection, which can be serious in the elderly. Notify the charge nurse in a timely manner.

ANSWER: b

Rationale:
Notify the nurse immediately if a client has a coffee-ground emesis. This is significant because it may indicate internal bleeding.

Basic Nursing Skills:
Data Collection and Reporting

18. **After the nurse aide measures the client's urinary output, he or she should:**

a. disinfect the graduate pitcher.

b. wipe the catheter tubing with alcohol.

c. provide perineal care.

d. store the graduate pitcher in a sealed container.

Answer ➡

Basic Nursing Skills:
Data Collection and Reporting

20. **Mr. King's vital signs are: temperature 100.7, taken rectally; pulse 96, respirations 18, blood pressure 128/74. How would the nurse aide document these findings?**

a. 100.7-18-96-128/74.

b. 96-18-128/74-100.7.

c. 100.7 (R)-96-18-128/74.

d. 100.7-96-18-128/74.

Answer ➡

Basic Nursing Skills:
Data Collection and Reporting

17. **The *primary* purpose of monitoring and recording urinary output is to:**

a. observe the color, character, and odor of the urine.

b. ensure that the urinary catheter is not obstructed.

c. ensure that the urinary catheter is emptied every shift.

d. ensure that the urinary output balances with the intake.

Answer ➡

Basic Nursing Skills:
Data Collection and Reporting

19. **The tympanic thermometer is used to measure temperature in the client's:**

a. mouth.

b. axilla.

c. rectum.

d. ear.

Answer ➡

ANSWER: a

Rationale:
Disinfect the graduate pitcher and allow it to dry thoroughly before storing it.

ANSWER: c

Rationale:
Record the method by which the temperature was taken. 100.7 (R) denotes that the temperature was taken rectally. Vital signs are recorded in this order: temperature, pulse, respiration, blood pressure.

ANSWER: d

Rationale:
The oral intake and urinary output should balance each day. The urinary output is slightly less than the fluid intake because the body uses some of the fluid each day. If the proper urinary balance is not maintained, the client may develop serious medical problems.

ANSWER: d

Rationale:
The tympanic temperature is the temperature taken at the tympanic membrane, in the ear.

Basic Nursing Skills:
Data Collection and Reporting

22. **You are assigned to take Mr. Brodsky's temperature rectally. Your facility uses color-coded glass thermometers. Which thermometer will you select?**

    a. The one with the blue dot on the end.

    b. The one with the green dot on the end.

    c. The one with the orange dot on the end.

    d. The one with the red dot on the end.

Answer ➤

Basic Nursing Skills:
Data Collection and Reporting

24. **Miss Nicoll is a confused, combative client who uses oxygen. She has a colostomy. You have been assigned to take her temperature. You will use the:**

    a. oral method.

    b. rectal method.

    c. electronic method.

    d. axillary method.

Answer ➤

Basic Nursing Skills:
Data Collection and Reporting

21. **You are assigned to take Mrs. Mangraviti's temperature by the axillary method. Your facility uses glass thermometers. Which thermometer will you use?**

    a. Oral.

    b. Rectal.

    c. Tympanic.

    d. Aural.

Answer ➤

Basic Nursing Skills:
Data Collection and Reporting

23. **Each long line on the glass thermometer denotes:**

    a. 1/10 degree.

    b. 2/10 degree.

    c. 1/8 degree.

    d. 1 degree.

Answer ➤

ANSWER: d

Rationale:
The rectal thermometer is always marked with a red marking.

ANSWER: a

Rationale:
Use an oral thermometer for taking an axillary temperature.

ANSWER: d

Rationale:
The client's confusion and combativeness make her a candidate for a rectal or axillary temperature. However, you cannot use the rectal method because of the colostomy. The only means available is the axillary method.

ANSWER: b

Rationale:
Each long line indicates 2/10 degree.

25. Of the methods listed for taking a temperature, which is the *least* accurate?

    a. Tympanic.

    b. Rectal.

    c. Axillary.

    d. Oral.

Answer ➥

---

26. The blood vessels that carry oxygen-rich blood to the various parts of the body are the:

    a. arteries.

    b. venules.

    c. veins.

    d. alveoli.

Answer ➥

---

27. Measure the blood pressure by placing the stethoscope over a:

    a. capillary.

    b. artery.

    c. venule.

    d. vein.

Answer ➥

---

28. The radial pulse is taken at the:

    a. neck.

    b. heart.

    c. bend of the elbow.

    d. wrist.

Answer ➥

ANSWER: a

Rationale:
The arteries carry freshly oxygenated blood to the various parts of the body.

ANSWER: c

Rationale:
The axillary method is the least accurate method of taking a temperature and should not be used if other methods are available.

ANSWER: d

Rationale:
The radial pulse is taken at the wrist.

ANSWER: b

Rationale:
Blood pressure is measured by placing a stethoscope over an artery.

Basic Nursing Skills:
Data Collection and Reporting

29. **The blood pressure is taken using the:**

a. carotid artery.

b. radial artery.

c. brachial artery.

d. femoral artery.

Answer ➥

Basic Nursing Skills:
Data Collection and Reporting

30. **Mr. Eliopoulos has an irregular pulse. You should count it for:**

a. one full minute.

b. five minutes.

c. 15 seconds.

d. 30 seconds.

Answer ➥

Basic Nursing Skills:
Data Collection and Reporting

31. **Mrs. McCloskey's pulse is strong and regular. To measure her pulse accurately, you should count for:**

a. 10 seconds, then multiply times 5.

b. 15 seconds, then multiply times 4.

c. 30 seconds, then multiply times 2.

d. 60 seconds, then multiply times 2.

Answer ➥

Basic Nursing Skills:
Data Collection and Reporting

32. **The *primary* purpose of the respiratory system is to:**

a. stimulate the heartbeat.

b. supply oxygen and eliminate carbon dioxide.

c. supply carbon dioxide and eliminate oxygen.

d. supply oxygen and eliminate carbon monoxide.

Answer ➥

ANSWER: a

Rationale:
If the pulse is irregular, check it for one full minute. Report your findings and observations to the charge nurse.

ANSWER: c

Rationale:
The brachial artery is used for checking blood pressure.

ANSWER: b

Rationale:
The primary purpose of the respiratory system is to supply oxygen and eliminate carbon dioxide from the body.

ANSWER: c

Rationale:
Because the client's pulse is regular, you may count for 30 seconds, then multiply times 2.

Basic Nursing Skills:
Data Collection and Reporting

34. **Mr. Matassarin was mentally alert yesterday. Today, when you enter his room to make the bed, he is very confused. His skin is flushed and he confides in you that he "doesn't feel good." You should:**

   a. give Mr. Matassarin a drink of cold water.

   b. make the bed and leave the room.

   c. report the change in condition to the nurse.

   d. put the client back to bed.

Answer ➨

Notes

Basic Nursing Skills:
Data Collection and Reporting

33. **To count respirations, the nurse aide should:**

   a. count one inhalation and one exhalation as one respiration.

   b. count one inhalation and one exhalation as two respirations.

   c. count only the exhaled breaths.

   d. divide the pulse rate by the number of breaths in a minute.

Answer ➨

Notes

ANSWER: c

Rationale:
Change in mental status is often significant in the elderly. Report the change in condition and your observations to the nurse in charge and follow his or her instructions for further care.

ANSWER: a

Rationale:
One inhalation and one exhalation equals one respiration.

Restorative Services: Prevention

2. **You must reposition a 90-pound, bedfast client on her left side. You should:**

   a. cross her legs at the ankles.

   b. place a pillow or thin pad between her lower legs.

   c. elevate the head of the bed.

   d. elevate the knee rest for comfort.

Answer ➡

Restorative Services: Prevention

4. **To prevent pressure ulcers, the nurse aide should turn and reposition the client in bed:**

   a. every 2 hours.

   b. every 3 hours.

   c. every 4 hours.

   d. once every shift.

Answer ➡

Restorative Services: Prevention

1. **You are assigned to ambulate a client who has a weak right side. For safety, you should apply a gait belt and stand:**

   a. on the client's right side.

   b. on the client's left side.

   c. in front of the client.

   d. behind the client.

Answer ➡

Restorative Services: Prevention

3. **A client has an abrasion on her coccyx. A common cause of this type of injury can be prevented by:**

   a. avoiding wrinkles in the sheets.

   b. padding the bed well.

   c. making sure there are no crumbs in the bed.

   d. avoiding friction and shear when pulling the client up in bed.

Answer ➡

ANSWER: b

Rationale:
Place a pillow or pad between the lower legs to prevent friction on the bony prominences, thus preventing pressure ulcers.

ANSWER: a

Rationale:
The client should be turned and repositioned every 2 hours, or more often if necessary to meet the client's individual needs.

ANSWER: a

Rationale:
Ambulation means to walk. Because the client's right side is weakest, stand on the right side. Grasp the center back of the gait belt firmly to ambulate the client.

ANSWER: d

Rationale:
An abrasion is like a burn that is caused by the friction of dragging the skin across the surface of the sheets.

Restorative Services: Prevention

6. To prevent external rotation of the hip in a bedfast client, the nurse aide should:

a. apply heel protectors.

b. support the leg with a trochanter roll.

c. place a pillow behind the client's back.

d. elevate the foot of the bed.

Answer ➔

Restorative Services: Prevention

8. Mr. Levitt had a stroke and has a weak left arm and leg. Which of these is the *best* method for preventing falls when transferring this client from bed to chair?

a. Move the client toward the weakest side.

b. Position the chair facing the bed and lock the brakes.

c. Use a transfer belt and move the client toward the strong side.

d. Lift Mr. Levitt; do not allow him to bear weight.

Answer ➔

Restorative Services: Prevention

5. The best method of preventing contractures is to:

a. reposition the client in bed at least hourly.

b. bathe the client twice a day.

c. provide range-of-motion exercises.

d. massage the skin with lotion every shift.

Answer ➔

Restorative Services: Prevention

7. Foot drop is a type of:

a. contracture.

b. pressure ulcer.

c. injury.

d. edema.

Answer ➔

ANSWER: b

Rationale:
A trochanter roll is used to support the leg and keep it from rotating outward.

ANSWER: c

Rationale:
Range-of-motion exercises involve taking each joint through its normal range of motion. This is the best method of preventing joint stiffening and muscle contractures.

ANSWER: c

Rationale:
Of the methods listed, the best is to apply a transfer belt. Position the chair so the client moves toward the strong side. Support the client with the transfer belt. Lock the brakes to the wheelchair during the transfer.

ANSWER: a

Rationale:
Foot drop is a contracture that can be prevented by using a footboard or adaptive footwear when the client is in bed.

Restorative Services: Prevention

9. **To prevent a flexion contracture of a paralyzed client's hand, the nurse aide should:**

   a. soak the hand in warm water twice a day.

   b. position a book or other object in the palm of the hand.

   c. apply a sling to the affected arm.

   d. place a handroll in the client's palm.

Answer ➥

Restorative Services: Prevention

10. **The purpose of a bed cradle is to:**

    a. keep the weight of the bedding off the client's skin.

    b. prevent contractures of the feet and legs.

    c. keep the restless client in bed.

    d. reduce the risk of edema.

Answer ➥

Restorative Services: Prevention

11. **The purpose of a footboard is to:**

    a. prevent edema of the feet and ankles.

    b. reduce the risk of pressure ulcers of the ankles and knees.

    c. enable the client to move the feet freely.

    d. prevent foot drop.

Answer ➥

Restorative Services: Prevention

12. **Miss Crenshaw is at high risk for pressure ulcers. She sits up in a wheelchair much of the day. The nurse aide should:**

    a. encourage her to stay in bed.

    b. apply a foam cushion to the chair.

    c. have her sit on a pillow.

    d. fold a sheet and place it on the seat of the chair.

Answer ➥

ANSWER: a

Rationale:
The bed cradle is used to keep the weight of the bed linen off the client's skin. A bed cradle is used for clients with many different skin conditions and burns, to keep the linen from sticking to ulcerated or injured areas. It is also used with some clients to prevent pressure and discomfort. A secondary effect is that it keeps the linen from pushing the client's feet downward, reducing the risk of foot drop.

ANSWER: d

Rationale:
A handroll is an effective method of preventing flexion contracture. A commercial handroll works best. Avoid using a rolled washcloth. The texture of the washcloth promotes squeezing, which may worsen the flexion.

ANSWER: b

Rationale:
Of the methods listed, placing a foam cushion in the seat of the chair is the best method of reducing pressure.

ANSWER: d

Rationale:
A footboard is placed at the foot of the bed to prevent foot drop, a serious contracture of the feet.

Restorative Services: Prevention

13. Mr. Bunton is a bedfast client with a stage IV pressure ulcer. He uses a therapeutic air mattress. The bottom sheet slides around on the mattress and gets bunched up under the client at least once a day. You should:

a. check the sheet frequently and straighten it when needed.

b. pin the sheet securely to the mattress.

c. tuck the sheet in very tightly.

d. tie the sheet to the side rails.

Answer →

Restorative Services: Prevention

14. Which of the following *do not* contribute to pressure ulcer development?

a. Adequate nutrition and hydration.

b. Pressure and friction.

c. Prolonged moisture.

d. Exposure to excretions.

Answer →

Restorative Services: Prevention

15. You are assigned to assist Mr. Frisch with passive range of motion. His elbow and knee joints are very stiff. You should:

a. apply firm pressure to bend the joints as far back as they will go.

b. move each joint gently, smoothly, and slowly.

c. quickly move each joint back and forth four times.

d. notify the nurse in charge immediately.

Answer →

Restorative Services: Prevention

16. Mrs. Hitchcock has an abrasion on her coccyx and a large red area on her left shoulder. You reposition her, but the redness does not go away. You should:

a. give her a good backrub, massaging both areas well.

b. apply alcohol to her back.

c. notify the nurse in charge.

d. apply a bandage to both areas.

Answer →

ANSWER: a

Rationale:
Of the choices listed, only "a" does not contribute to pressure ulcer development.

ANSWER: a

Rationale:
Never use pins when an air mattress is in use. Tucking the sheet in tightly may restrict air flow, defeating the purpose of the mattress. Of the answers listed here, the best is to check the client frequently and straighten the sheet as often as needed.

ANSWER: c

Rationale:
The appearance of both areas suggests that they are developing pressure ulcers. Avoid rubbing the areas, which may worsen tissue damage. Do not apply any products to the areas. Notify the nurse of your observations.

ANSWER: b

Rationale:
Move each joint gently, slowly, and smoothly at least 5 times, or according to facility policy. Avoid forcing the joint past the point of pain or resistance.

Restorative Services: Prevention

18. Mrs. Paquette had a stroke and is at risk of contractures. The occupational therapist fabricated a hand and wrist splint for her to wear during the day. The splint is removed at bedtime. The nurse aide should:

a. never remove the splint, as this is the nurse's responsibility.

b. keep the hand clean and dry under the splint.

c. always elevate the client's splinted hand on a pillow.

d. support the splinted extremity with a sling.

Answer ➜

Notes

Restorative Services: Prevention

17. Contractures are:

a. relaxation and extension of muscles.

b. tremors.

c. normal in aging.

d. shortening and stiffening of muscles.

Answer ➜

Restorative Services: Prevention

19. Before applying Mrs. Paquette's splint, the nurse aide should:

a. consult the care plan for instructions.

b. ask the client's daughter how to apply the splint.

c. wash the splint in warm, running water.

d. wrap the hand lightly with a bandage.

Answer ➜

ANSWER: b

Rationale:
The nurse aide is responsible for keeping a splinted extremity clean and dry.

ANSWER: d

Rationale:
Contractures are deformities caused by shortening and stiffening of muscles from lack of use.

ANSWER: a

Rationale:
If the nurse aide is not familiar with the splinting procedure, he or she should consult the care plan for specific instructions.

Restorative Services: Self Care/Independence

2. **A mentally alert, talkative client has quadriplegia and cannot care for himself because his arms and legs are paralyzed. Promote positive self-esteem and participation in his care by:**

a. giving him choices and asking his opinion and preferences in daily routines.

b. setting up supplies and directing him to use them, as a means of testing his ability.

c. treating him like your equal and discussing your personal life with him.

d. saying as little as possible so you do not upset the client.

Answer ➡

Restorative Services: Self Care/Independence

4. **A client with Alzheimer's disease wanders aimlessly about the facility. She is incontinent several times daily on your shift. The best way to assist this client to maintain her independence and dignity by:**

a. dressing her in an incontinence brief so her clothes do not get wet.

b. reminding her to use the bathroom when you pass her in the hall.

c. taking her to the bathroom every 2 to 3 hours during your shift.

d. providing incontinent care as often as necessary each day.

Answer ➡

Restorative Services: Self Care/Independence

1. **You are assigned to bathe a confused client who talks a great deal, but does not make sense. She responds appropriately part of the time. The assignment sheet says she can wash her upper body. Another nurse aide tells you the client is very slow and needs total care. You should:**

a. provide a complete bath based on the information given by the other nurse aide.

b. set up the supplies and see how the client responds when asked to wash her face.

c. bathe the client completely, because doing so is faster.

d. skip the bath for today, because bathing the client is too confusing.

Answer ➡

Restorative Services: Self Care/Independence

3. **A client with a right arm injury is very frustrated because he cannot use his right hand. He tells you that he cannot feed himself. Your best response is:**

a. "Yes, you can."

b. "I will feed you."

c. "You can't use your right hand; you must use your left."

d. "You can use your left hand. I'll help if you have trouble."

Answer ➡

ANSWER: a

Rationale:
Avoid testing the client's self-care ability. His self-esteem will be enhanced if he has as much control over his environment and routines as possible. Giving him choices of clothing, time to do activities, and so on will have a positive effect.

ANSWER: b

Rationale:
The client has the potential to bathe herself. Because you are not familiar with her, set up the supplies and give her directions to see how she responds. If successful, give her another direction. Avoid giving too many directions at one time, as this may overwhelm or confuse her.

ANSWER: c

Rationale:
Of the answers given, the best is "c." Regular toileting is the best way to prevent incontinence in a confused client who cannot determine her own needs.

ANSWER: d

Rationale:
A principle of restorative nursing is to stress the client's ability, not the disability. In keeping with this philosophy, "d" is the best answer. It stresses the client's remaining ability, but also advises that you are willing to help if need be.

Restorative Services:
Self Care/Independence

6. **Restorative nursing care is designed to:**

a. be given only by licensed personnel.

b. require the skills of a therapist.

c. maintain or improve clients.

d. promote dependence in ADLs.

Answer ➥

Restorative Services:
Self Care/Independence

8. **You are assisting a client with a restorative bathing program. He becomes impatient when he can't squeeze the water out of the washcloth. The *best* thing to do is:**

a. use hand-over-hand technique.

b. squeeze the water out of the washcloth and wash his face.

c. allow the client to struggle slightly, but not to the point of frustration.

d. tell the client that he can try again another day.

Answer ➥

Restorative Services:
Self Care/Independence

5. **Clients with a disability may be able to be more independent if:**

a. the nurse aide gives them plenty of encouragement.

b. they learn how to use adaptive devices to make ADLs easier.

c. they exercise the affected body part each day.

d. the doctor prescribes more medication.

Answer ➥

Restorative Services:
Self Care/Independence

7. **Mrs. Li had a stroke and is paralyzed on the right side of her body. She becomes frustrated when she feeds herself. She scoops the food onto a spoon. As she does this, the plate slides away from her on the table. The *best* way for the nurse aide to help Mrs. Li is to:**

a. place a wet washcloth or piece of gripper under her plate.

b. spoon-feed her to decrease her anxiety.

c. apply an adaptive plate guard for her dinner plate.

d. place a napkin under her plate.

Answer ➥

ANSWER: c

Rationale:
The OBRA nursing home laws require facilities to maintain or improve clients unless this is medically impossible. Restorative nursing care is basic nursing care that is designed to maintain or improve client ability.

ANSWER: c

Rationale:
Allowing the client to struggle slightly will help him overcome the disability. However, you must not allow him to become too frustrated and upset. If he struggles and still cannot remove the water, pick up the washcloth, squeeze the excess water out, then hand it back to the client so he can finish the task.

ANSWER: b

Rationale:
Adaptive devices are pieces of equipment designed to make everyday tasks easier for individuals with specific disabilities. The nurse aide can help teach clients how to use adaptive devices and encourage them when they begin doing so. The teaching, praise, and encouragement promote client independence.

ANSWER: a

Rationale:
A wet washcloth or piece of gripper (dycem) under the plate will hold it in place on the table and prevent sliding.

Restorative Services:
Self Care/Independence

10. **A client who is on a bowel and bladder retraining program:**

   a. is taken to the bathroom routinely every 2 hours.

   b. is toileted on an assessment-based schedule.

   c. should have his or her fluid intake limited.

   d. must be awakened every hour during the night to check for incontinence.

Answer ➥

Notes

Restorative Services:
Self Care/Independence

9. **Inactivity and immobility:**

   a. are important for clients who are ill.

   b. are the norm for long-term care clients.

   c. can cause weakness and muscle wasting.

   d. cause the client to become strong and healthy.

Answer ➥

Notes

ANSWER: b

Rationale:
Bowel and bladder retraining is an assessment-based program developed by the nurse on an individualized schedule. Toileting every 2 hours is not considered an active retraining program.

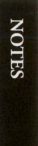

ANSWER: c

Rationale:
Inactivity and immobility are not good for most people. They cause many complications, including weakness and muscle wasting. All clients should be encouraged to be as active as possible each day.

Psychosocial Care Skills: Emotional and Mental Health Needs

1. You enter the room to give AM care and find Mrs. Tucker crying. Your best response is to:

   a. quietly leave the room, closing the door behind you.

   b. ask the client if she wants to talk about what is bothering her.

   c. notify the nurse in charge immediately.

   d. tell Mrs. Tucker that everything will be all right.

Answer ➥

Psychosocial Care Skills: Emotional and Mental Health Needs

2. Mr. Rizzo, a client with Alzheimer's disease, tells you that he is leaving to go to work now. Your best response is:

   a. "You haven't worked in years."

   b. "You cannot leave."

   c. "That will be fine."

   d. "Tell me about your work."

Answer ➥

Psychosocial Care Skills: Emotional and Mental Health Needs

3. A confused client screams and tries to hit you when you bathe her. You understand that:

   a. the client does not like you.

   b. the client does not want you to care for her.

   c. she is communicating through her behavior.

   d. the client prefers a shower.

Answer ➥

Psychosocial Care Skills: Emotional and Mental Health Needs

4. Self-esteem is:

   a. feeling important and worthwhile.

   b. need for love.

   c. a need for safety.

   d. feeling as if one belongs to a certain group.

Answer ➥

ANSWER: d

Rationale:
A client who says he is going to work is looking for a state of mind, not a physical location. Do not argue with him about his job. He will not believe you. The best approach to take is to ask him about his job. Speaking about it will help him restore the state of mind he is seeking.

ANSWER: b

Rationale:
Before taking further action, the best action is to find out what is troubling the client. Ask her to tell you what is wrong and allow her to talk about it. Avoid giving her false hope.

ANSWER: a

Rationale:
Self-esteem is a need of all people. Everyone has a need to feel important and worthwhile. The nurse aide must promote positive self-esteem for the clients.

ANSWER: c

Rationale:
The client has lost her ability for meaningful communication. Do not take the behavior personally. Screaming and hitting may be the only method she has of expressing her displeasure.

Psychosocial Care Skills: Emotional and Mental Health Needs

6. A developmental task that aging clients must work through is:

   a. trusting others.

   b. developing a sense of identity.

   c. review of life events.

   d. developing a sense of initiative.

Answer →

Psychosocial Care Skills: Emotional and Mental Health Needs

8. A dying client is angry and tells you, "This food isn't fit for a dog." Your best response is:

   a. "It's the same thing we have every Monday."

   b. "Everyone else is eating it without complaining."

   c. "I'll see if I can find something else for you."

   d. "You don't have to eat it if you don't like it."

Answer →

Psychosocial Care Skills: Emotional and Mental Health Needs

5. A client has had a breast removed because of cancer. When she returns, she tells you, "I look so ugly." Your best response is:

   a. "You'll feel better in a few weeks."

   b. "You shouldn't feel so sorry for yourself."

   c. "I will get the nurse."

   d. "I don't think you are ugly at all."

Answer →

Psychosocial Care Skills: Emotional and Mental Health Needs

7. A dying client says, "If only God will spare me this, I'll go to Mass every week." Your best response is:

   a. "I go to church weekly."

   b. "Would you like a visit from your priest?"

   c. "I'll tell the nurse to call your daughter."

   d. "Everything will be just fine."

Answer →

ANSWER: c

Rationale:
The elderly review life events and circumstances, developing feelings of acceptance, fulfillment, and self-worth.

ANSWER: d

Rationale:
Telling the client how you feel about her will help her feel better about herself. Giving her a hug may also be appropriate.

ANSWER: c

Rationale:
The client is grieving and needs your understanding and support. Try to meet reasonable needs and demands for a different selection promptly.

ANSWER: b

Rationale:
Responding to the client is difficult in this situation. The client is in the bargaining stage of the grieving process. Because she is thinking about religion, she may appreciate a visit from her clergyperson.

10. Mrs. Stone is a confused client. When you enter her room with her breakfast tray, she is removing her clothes. She says, "I'm getting ready for bed now." To orient her to reality, your best response is:

    a. "It is not bedtime."

    b. "It is 8:00 A.M. Would you like some breakfast?"

    c. "Please put your clothes back on."

    d. "No, don't do that. It's morning. You just got up."

Answer ➡

12. Reminiscence is an activity used for assisting clients who are mentally confused. When using this technique, the nurse aide helps the client to:

    a. remember the past.

    b. orient to reality.

    c. validate his or her feelings.

    d. perform activities.

Answer ➡

9. A newly admitted client yells at you when you enter the room. She tells you she wants to go home. Help her adjust to living in the nursing facility by:

    a. giving her choices and control.

    b. setting strict routines.

    c. providing total care.

    d. telling her things will get better.

Answer ➡

11. A client has been told that she is dying. She tells you, "They are wrong. I don't feel sick." You know that she is experiencing:

    a. bargaining.

    b. anger.

    c. denial.

    d. acceptance.

Answer ➡

ANSWER: b

Rationale:
Of the answers listed, "b" gives the client the time. It also tells her that you are bringing breakfast, a meal associated with morning time. If the client has a clock in the room, you may also call her attention to the time on the clock.

ANSWER: a

Rationale:
Newly admitted clients grieve for many losses, including their homes, belongings, and loss of physical function. Help the client by giving her choices about her routines, time of day to bathe, preferences in care, and so on. Giving her control is a good way of helping her adjust to life in the facility.

ANSWER: a

Rationale:
Reminiscence is a useful technique in which the client with cognitive impairment remembers and discusses events of the past.

ANSWER: c

Rationale:
The client is in denial, the first stage of the grieving process. In this stage, she does not accept or believe the diagnosis.

Psychosocial Care Skills: Emotional and Mental Health Needs

13. When using validation to assist a client with Alzheimer's, the nurse aide:

a. orients the client to reality.

b. uses puzzles and challenging activities.

c. uses music therapy.

d. encourages clients to express feelings.

Answer ➥

Psychosocial Care Skills: Emotional and Mental Health Needs

15. A client with dementia sits in her chair in the hallway screaming. She may be doing this because she:

a. is trying to be annoying.

b. is unhappy in the nursing home.

c. doesn't like the staff on duty.

d. has an unmet need.

Answer ➥

Psychosocial Care Skills: Emotional and Mental Health Needs

14. A client with Alzheimer's disease says she is going home to cook dinner for her children and starts out the door. The best approach to take with this client is to:

a. tell the client that her children are grown.

b. walk with her and ask what she likes to cook.

c. inform her it is too cold to go outside.

d. tell her the nursing facility is her home.

Answer ➥

Psychosocial Care Skills: Emotional and Mental Health Needs

16. A client disrobes in the hallway several times during your shift. You should:

a. scold her, then get her dressed.

b. remind her that her behavior is not appropriate.

c. dress her, then tell her how nice she looks.

d. ignore the behavior.

Answer ➥

ANSWER: b

Rationale:
Walk with the client and talk to her about cooking to restore the state of mind she is seeking. Ask her how to prepare her favorite dishes. Circle back into the facility. Telling her not to go out or that the facility is her home is likely to cause agitation. Avoid arguing with the client.

ANSWER: c

Rationale:
Scolding the client will not work. Behavior that is rewarded by attention is likely to be repeated. Dress the client, then compliment her on her appearance.

ANSWER: d

Rationale:
Validation helps clients regain feelings of dignity and self-control by validating their feelings.

ANSWER: d

Rationale:
Clients with dementia often act out because of basic needs that are not met, such as hunger, thirst, pain, or need to use the bathroom. If the need is met, the behavior stops.

Psychosocial Care Skills: Emotional and Mental Health Needs

18. Mr. Strong yells and tells you he is very angry with you because he cannot find his favorite sweater. You know that:

a. someone lost his sweater.

b. he is angry with his situation.

c. he is very angry with you.

d. the client is confused.

Answer ➥

Psychosocial Care Skills: Emotional and Mental Health Needs

20. You knock on Mr. Crenshaw's door, but there is no answer. You crack the door and look into the room. The client is in bed with his wife. You should:

a. close the door and leave them alone.

b. advise them that visiting hours are over.

c. tell them to stop acting like children.

d. inform the nurse in charge immediately.

Answer ➥

Psychosocial Care Skills: Emotional and Mental Health Needs

17. A client with dementia is wandering into other clients' rooms. He tells you he is looking for the bathroom. You should:

a. take him to the bathroom and assist him as needed.

b. tell him to go to his own room to use the bathroom.

c. tell him how to find the bathroom.

d. advise him not to go in other clients' rooms.

Answer ➥

Psychosocial Care Skills: Emotional and Mental Health Needs

19. Mrs. Dibbles is sitting in her wheelchair masturbating in the hallway. The nurse aide should:

a. tell the client to stop acting like a fool.

b. instruct her to go to her room.

c. take her to her room and provide privacy.

d. ignore her and say nothing.

Answer ➥

ANSWER: b

Rationale:
The nurse aide will probably have to modify his or her behavior in response to the client's behavior. The client is not angry with you. You are the first person he saw and he struck out. He is angry with his situation. Help him find his sweater, if possible. Avoid verbally striking back.

ANSWER: a

Rationale:
The client has dementia and will not be able to remember or follow your instructions. Taking him to the bathroom is the most effective approach.

ANSWER: a

Rationale:
Elderly individuals have the same sexual needs as younger adults. Close the door and leave the room.

ANSWER: c

Rationale:
The best action to take is to push her wheelchair to her room. Assist her to bed if necessary or desired. Provide privacy and leave the room.

Psychosocial Care Skills: Emotional and Mental Health Needs

22. Mr. Bradigan is scheduled for a shower today. Facility activities are scheduled for 10:00 and 2:00. You know that Mr. Bradigan enjoys the current-events class at 10:00. You should:

a. assume that the client will attend current events if he wants to go.

b. remind him of the activity and ask if he wants his shower early.

c. inform him that you plan to shower him at 10:00 so he cannot attend.

d. not mention the activity, so that he will not disrupt your routine.

Answer ☛

Notes

Psychosocial Care Skills: Emotional and Mental Health Needs

21. It is time for Mrs. Heaney's shower. She tells you she does not want a shower. She says she wants to go to the Bingo activity right now. You should:

a. insist that she take a shower.

b. tell her she cannot go to Bingo until she showers.

c. arrange to shower her after she returns from Bingo.

d. ask the nurse in charge what to do.

Answer ☛

Notes

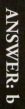

ANSWER: b

Rationale:
Modify your routine to meet the client's needs. Arrange to shower the client before the activity so he can attend.

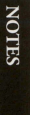

NOTES

ANSWER: c

Rationale:
The client has the right to set her own schedule. Allow her to go to Bingo and rearrange your schedule so you can shower her when she returns.

NOTES

Psychosocial Care Skills: Spiritual and Cultural Needs

1. **Culture is:**

   a. a religious belief.

   b. an improper ethic or standard.

   c. a pattern or lifestyle.

   d. a judgment.

Answer →

Psychosocial Care Skills: Spiritual and Cultural Needs

3. **Mrs. Duke tells you that her priest will be visiting at 10:00 to give her Communion. The nurse aide should:**

   a. do nothing, as the client is expecting the visit.

   b. inform her that 10:00 is time for her bath.

   c. ask if you can help her prepare for the visit.

   d. notify the social worker.

Answer →

Psychosocial Care Skills: Spiritual and Cultural Needs

2. **Mr. Weiss was admitted several days ago. You notice that he never drinks the milk on his supper tray, although he usually eats the rest of his meal. One day you ask him if he doesn't like milk. He informs you that his religion prohibits him from having milk and meat together. You should:**

   a. do nothing, as this is his choice.

   b. notify the nurse that he needs a different beverage.

   c. offer him a can of supplement in place of the milk.

   d. document that he refused the milk.

Answer →

Psychosocial Care Skills: Spiritual and Cultural Needs

4. **When the priest arrives, you are making Mrs. Duke's roommate's bed. You should:**

   a. provide privacy for the client and priest.

   b. ask the priest to wait in the lounge until you are done.

   c. visit with the priest while you are making the bed.

   d. inform the nurse that you cannot complete your work.

Answer →

ANSWER: b

Rationale:
Notify the nurse or other appropriate person that the client is not drinking the milk for religious reasons. The nurse can arrange for the client to get a different beverage with his meals.

ANSWER: c

Rationale:
Culture is the pattern or lifestyle of a group of people. Culture affects many health care practices and beliefs. Avoid stereotyping others who are from a different culture than your own. Respect their practices and beliefs.

ANSWER: a

Rationale:
Provide privacy for the client and priest by pulling the privacy curtain, or leaving the room, as appropriate. If you must leave the roommate's bed unmade, return later to complete the task.

ANSWER: c

Rationale:
The client is expecting this visit. Arrange to bathe and dress her early. Help her with any special preparations.

Role of the Nurse Aide: Communication

2. **The nurse aide should approach a client with Alzheimer's disease from the:**

   a. left side.

   b. right side.

   c. front.

   d. rear.

Answer ➥

Role of the Nurse Aide: Communication

4. **When caring for a client who is blind, the nurse aide should avoid:**

   a. speaking.

   b. rapid movements.

   c. words like "see," "hear," and "go."

   d. rearranging the client's belongings.

Answer ➥

Role of the Nurse Aide: Communication

1. **When entering the room of a client who is blind, the nurse aide should:**

   a. greet the client by name and introduce himself or herself.

   b. be as quiet as possible so as not to disturb the client.

   c. speak loudly into the client's ear.

   d. go about his or her business as if the client were not there.

Answer ➥

Role of the Nurse Aide: Communication

3. **To communicate with a client who is hard of hearing, the nurse aide should:**

   a. yell loudly into the client's ear.

   b. face the client and make sure he or she can see the aide's face.

   c. always use sign language.

   d. write everything on a piece of paper.

Answer ➥

ANSWER: c

Rationale:
Approach the client from the front so he or she can see you. Approaching from the sides or rear may startle the client, causing him or her to have a catastrophic reaction.

ANSWER: d

Rationale:
Avoid rearranging things in the client's room. If you move the client's belongings, he or she will be unable to find them. Words like "see" are acceptable in conversation.

ANSWER: a

Rationale:
Because the client cannot see you, he or she will not know you are there unless you introduce yourself. Tell the client who you are and what you plan to do.

ANSWER: b

Rationale:
Clients who are hard of hearing usually do not speak sign language, as many hearing losses develop late in life. Most communicate verbally. Face the client. Speak slowly and distinctly.

Role of the Nurse Aide: Communication

5. When walking with a client who is blind:

a. hold the upper arm lightly and walk slightly ahead of the client.

b. stand in front of the client and take him or her by the hand.

c. be as silent as possible so the client can focus on the ambulation.

d. always avoid stairs or uneven surfaces.

Answer ➔

Role of the Nurse Aide: Communication

6. Touching clients:

a. is always offensive.

b. should be avoided if possible.

c. communicates that you care.

d. is a sexual gesture.

Answer ➔

Role of the Nurse Aide: Communication

7. Listening is:

a. a form of communication.

b. not important to the elderly.

c. sometimes offensive.

d. not a nurse aide skill.

Answer ➔

Role of the Nurse Aide: Communication

8. The nurse aide's body language:

a. is not important to the client.

b. is a form of communication.

c. should be very still.

d. should be stiff and rigid.

Answer ➔

ANSWER: c

Rationale:
All humans need to be touched, but use good judgment about touching clients. Avoid startling an agitated client. In general, lightly touching the forearm or hand communicates that you care and is therapeutic.

ANSWER: a

Rationale:
When walking with a blind client, grasp the upper arm lightly and walk slightly ahead of the client. Tell him or her about obstacles, turns, and uneven surfaces.

ANSWER: b

o

Rationale:
Body language is a form of communication. Monitor your body language for the message it sends to the client.

ANSWER: a

Rationale:
Listening is an important form of communication. The nurse aide must listen to the clients, to supervisors, to coworkers, and to others.

Role of the Nurse Aide: Communication

10. Mr. Wright's son complains that the previous shift left his father wet. Your best response is:

a. "I will tell them not to do it again."

b. "I understand why you are upset. I'll tell the nurse."

c. "They were short of staff today."

d. "We are having some trouble with the staff on that shift."

Answer ➜

Notes

Role of the Nurse Aide: Communication

9. Mrs. Delgado's daughter asks you what's wrong with the client in room 213. Your best response is:

a. "She has cancer."

b. "I'm not supposed to tell you, but she has renal failure."

c. "I cannot discuss the other clients. You need to speak with the nurse."

d. "It's none of your business."

Answer ➜

Role of the Nurse Aide: Communication

11. When passing family members and visitors in the hallway, the nurse aide should:

a. be as silent as possible.

b. quickly look the other way.

c. pretend to be busy.

d. smile and greet the visitors.

Answer ➜

ANSWER: b

Rationale:
Your best response is to validate the family member's concerns by acknowledging that you think they are legitimate. Informing the client that you will report to the nurse indicates that the complaint will be followed up. Avoid discussing staffing problems with clients' family members.

NOTES

ANSWER: c

Rationale:
Tactfully inform the daughter that you cannot disclose information about other clients. Direct her to the nurse in charge.

ANSWER: d

Rationale:
Always smile, speak to, and welcome visitors to your facility.

Role of the Nurse Aide:
Client Rights

2. **Mr. Parker must be spoon-fed. He eats very slowly. Your unit is busy. You observe another nurse aide flushing Mr. Parker's meal down the commode. Failing to feed a client is an example of:**

   a. abuse.

   b. neglect.

   c. libel.

   d. defamation.

Answer ➡

Role of the Nurse Aide:
Client Rights

4. **You witness another employee eating candy from a box in the client's drawer. The employee empties the box, closes the lid, and leaves it in the drawer. This is an example of:**

   a. abuse.

   b. neglect.

   c. mistreatment of property.

   d. misappropriation of property.

Answer ➡

Role of the Nurse Aide:
Client Rights

1. **You were off yesterday. When you return to work today, you notice bruises on a client's upper arms. You should:**

   a. call the police immediately.

   b. report your findings to the nurse in charge.

   c. tell the administrator that the client was abused.

   d. notify the client's daughter of the bruises.

Answer ➡

Role of the Nurse Aide:
Client Rights

3. **You observe another employee hitting a client. When your coworker notices you, he says he is having a bad day and asks you not to tell anyone. You should:**

   a. notify the nurse in charge.

   b. say nothing, as the employee is having a bad day.

   c. call the police.

   d. ask another nurse aide for advice.

Answer ➡

ANSWER: b

Rationale:
Deliberately or unintentionally failing to feed a client is neglect. Neglect is illegal and should be reported to the nurse in charge.

ANSWER: b

Rationale:
Report your observations to the nurse in charge. He or she will assess the client and take the appropriate action.

ANSWER: d

Rationale:
This is an example of misappropriation (taking) of property. Report your observations to the nurse in charge.

ANSWER: a

Rationale:
Do not discuss your observations with other employees. Report the situation to the nurse in charge. He or she will take the appropriate action.

Role of the Nurse Aide:
Client Rights

5. **You are assigned to give a client a bed bath. There is no one in the hallway and no one in the room with the client. You should:**

   a. leave the door to the room open, but pull the privacy curtain.

   b. close the door to the room, the window curtain, and privacy curtain.

   c. close the door to the room, but leave the window and privacy curtains open.

   d. ask the client if he wants you to leave the curtains open or closed.

Answer ➥

Role of the Nurse Aide:
Client Rights

6. **Miss Black tells you she has a bank account that she does not want her daughter to know about. You should:**

   a. report this information to the nurse in charge.

   b. tell the social worker.

   c. inform the client's daughter of the bank account.

   d. say nothing about this to anyone.

Answer ➥

Role of the Nurse Aide:
Client Rights

7. **Mrs. Bellai tells you that her husband has been hitting her. You should:**

   a. say nothing about this to anyone.

   b. tell the husband you will turn him in to the authorities if he does it again.

   c. notify the nurse in charge.

   d. call the police.

Answer ➥

Role of the Nurse Aide:
Client Rights

8. **You find a number of pills wrapped in tissue in a client's drawer. The client confides that she is not taking her medicine and asks you not to tell anyone. You should:**

   a. inform the client's family.

   b. remove the pills and notify the nurse.

   c. respect the client's confidence and say nothing.

   d. leave the pills and notify the administrator.

Answer ➥

ANSWER: d

Rationale:
The presence of a bank account does not affect the client's care. Say nothing to anyone and respect the client's confidence.

ANSWER: b

Rationale:
Always close the door to the room, privacy curtain, and window curtain when giving personal care or when the client's body is exposed.

ANSWER: b

Rationale:
Remove the pills from the client's room. They present a danger to the client and others. Inform the charge nurse.

ANSWER: c

Rationale:
Notify the nurse in charge of the client's complaint. Do not discuss the situation with anyone else.

Role of the Nurse Aide: Client Rights

9. State surveyors are in the facility. A client tells you that she complained to the surveyors about the nurse in charge of the unit. You should:

   a. inform the nurse of the client's complaint.

   b. notify the social worker.

   c. say nothing, as the client has the right to complain.

   d. inform the surveyors that the client is senile and should not be taken seriously.

Answer ➔

Role of the Nurse Aide: Client Rights

10. Mr. Papadakis is hard of hearing. He turns the volume up high on his television set. Several other clients complain about the noise. Your best response is to:

    a. do nothing, as the client has a right to turn the volume up as high as he wants.

    b. inform the client that the television is disturbing others and ask him to turn it down.

    c. go immediately to the client's room and turn the television off.

    d. notify the social worker of the problem.

Answer ➔

Role of the Nurse Aide: Client Rights

11. Mrs. Pagano informs you that she is voting for the Republican candidate in the election. You plan to vote for the Democratic candidate. You should:

    a. say nothing to the client, as she can vote for whomever she chooses.

    b. tell the client why the Democratic candidate is a better choice.

    c. tell her you will help fill out her ballot, then vote for the Democrat.

    d. notify the nurse in charge.

Answer ➔

Role of the Nurse Aide: Client Rights

12. Mrs. Szuchman tells you she wants to wear the blue blouse. You think the white blouse is prettier. You should:

    a. give the client the white blouse.

    b. give the client the blue blouse.

    c. tell her the blue blouse is dirty.

    d. pretend you cannot find the blue blouse.

Answer ➔

ANSWER: b

Rationale:
Ask the client to turn the television down. If this is a problem, notify the nurse in charge.

ANSWER: b

Rationale:
Give Mrs. Szuchman the blue blouse. She has the right to wear the clothing of her choice.

ANSWER: c

Rationale:
Clients have the right to complain to the survey agency without fear of reprisal. Keep the information confidential.

ANSWER: a

Rationale:
Clients have the right to make decisions and personal choices. Say nothing to the client about her choice of candidates.

Role of the Nurse Aide: Client Rights

13. Mr. Stone is very confused. You are assisting him with his ADLs. He often puts on clothing that does not match. When it is time to dress the client, you should:

a. open the closet and ask what he wants to wear.

b. select the clothing for the client.

c. ask if he wants to wear the red shirt or the blue shirt.

d. ask the nurse in charge what you should do.

Answer ➤

Role of the Nurse Aide: Client Rights

14. Mrs. Long has a $50 bill in her drawer. The nurse aide should:

a. give the money to the social worker.

b. ask the client to keep a smaller amount and store the rest in the safe.

c. do nothing, as the client has the right to keep the money.

d. inform the other nurse aides that the client has $50 in the drawer.

Answer ➤

Role of the Nurse Aide: Client Rights

15. Mr. Hegle is constantly leaving his dentures in the bed. He has two denture cups in his drawer. You know that the dentures will be ruined if they accidentally go through the washer and dryer. You should:

a. check the linen carefully for dentures before placing it in the wash.

b. do nothing, as the dentures are Mr. Hegle's responsibility.

c. notify the nurse in charge.

d. shake the linen out when removing it from the bed.

Answer ➤

Role of the Nurse Aide: Client Rights

16. Your unit is busy. A client keeps wandering into others' rooms, upsetting them. Another nurse aide suggests that you apply a restraint to keep the client from wandering. You should:

a. apply a vest restraint immediately.

b. place the client in a geriatric chair.

c. avoid using restraints without an order.

d. do nothing, as the client has a right to wander.

Answer ➤

ANSWER: b

Rationale:
Clients have the right to keep money. However, storing a large amount in an unlocked drawer is not safe. Try to talk the client into keeping a smaller amount and depositing the rest in her trust account or the facility safe. Say nothing about the money to the other nurse aides.

ANSWER: c

Rationale:
The client has the right to make choices even though he is confused. However, asking him to select his clothing from the closet may be overwhelming to him. Giving him limited choices respects his dignity and client rights.

ANSWER: c

Rationale:
The nurse aide should intervene. Restraints may not be used without a physician's order, or for staff convenience. However, the wanderer is upsetting other clients. Try to find an activity to occupy the wanderer without using restraints.

ANSWER: a

Rationale:
You must assist the client to safeguard his dentures. Check the linen carefully, but avoid shaking it, which spreads microbes in the air.

Role of the Nurse Aide:
Client Rights

17. **You are assigned to assist a new admission in storing her belongings. The client brought family pictures, a few knick-knacks, and a stuffed animal from home. You should:**

a. put all the client's belongings away in the closet and drawers.

b. inform the client that personal items collect dust and should not be used.

c. ask the client's daughter to take the personal items home.

d. assist the client to display her personal items in an attractive manner.

Answer ➡

Notes

Role of the Nurse Aide:
Client Rights

18. **A client asks you to read a letter to him. You should:**

a. tell him that the letter is personal and you cannot read it.

b. consult the nurse in charge.

c. read the letter to the client.

d. tell him you are too busy to read the letter.

Answer ➡

Notes

ANSWER: c

Rationale:
By asking you to read the letter, the client has waived his right to privacy. Assist him by reading the letter to him.

NOTES

ANSWER: d

Rationale:
Clients have the right to display important personal items. The nurse aide should assist the client in making her room comfortable and homelike.

NOTES

Role of the Nurse Aide:
Legal and Ethical Behavior

2. A confused client tells you that he does not want to take a shower. The client smells bad. Your best response is to:

a. honor the client's wishes, as he has the right to refuse.

b. force the client to take a shower.

c. notify the social worker immediately.

d. return later to see if the client will agree to the shower.

Answer ☛

Role of the Nurse Aide:
Legal and Ethical Behavior

4. The standard of care:

a. does not apply to nurse aides.

b. is a complicated medical concept.

c. is what a reasonable, prudent nurse aide would do in a similar situation.

d. is an administrative responsibility that does not apply to personal care.

Answer ☛

Role of the Nurse Aide:
Legal and Ethical Behavior

1. A mentally alert client tells you that she wants to die and is going to stop going to dialysis. The nurse, social worker, and client's daughter have been discussing this decision. You know that the:

a. client has the right to make health care decisions, but must be informed of the consequences of her decisions.

b. client cannot do this and that the client's daughter will force her to continue dialysis.

c. family will make all health care decisions.

d. doctor will not permit the client to stop dialysis.

Answer ☛

Role of the Nurse Aide:
Legal and Ethical Behavior

3. A client asks you questions about your personal life. You should:

a. tell him whatever he wants to know.

b. confide in him and ask advice about your personal problems.

c. give him general information, but avoid personal problems.

d. inform him that you cannot talk about your personal life.

Answer ☛

ANSWER: d

Rationale:
This is a difficult situation, but is commonly seen in health care. Bathing has an effect on the client's overall health. Other clients should not have to tolerate bad smells. If the client has a durable power of attorney for health care, that person makes the decisions, not the confused client. Your best approach in this situation is to avoid arguing with the client, then return again later and try again. He may agree to the shower when you return. If he continues to refuse, report it to the nurse in charge.

ANSWER: a

Rationale:
Mentally alert clients have the right to make decisions. However, they must be informed of the consequences of their decisions.

ANSWER: c

Rationale:
Standards of care are common, acceptable health care practice. Standards are defined by community, state, and national practices and involve what a reasonable, prudent nurse aide would do in the same or similar situation.

ANSWER: c

Rationale:
Talking about your interests, family, and other subjects is acceptable. Avoid talking to clients about personal problems.

Role of the Nurse Aide:
Legal and Ethical Behavior

5. **Mrs. Mangano has an order for a belt restraint in the wheelchair. She can also use the geriatric (geri) chair. When applying restraints to this client, the nurse aide should:**

a. use the least restrictive restraint for the least amount of time.

b. restrain the client in a wheelchair with a vest.

c. place the client in the geriatric chair.

d. apply the belt restraint in the geriatric chair.

Answer ☛

Notes

Notes

Notes

ANSWER: a

Rationale:
When there is a choice of restraints, always select the least restrictive device. If it is ineffective, use the more restrictive device.

Role of the Nurse Aide: Member of the Health Care Team

1. **The nurse aide's immediate supervisor is the:**

   a. director of nursing.

   b. administrator.

   c. charge nurse.

   d. coordinator.

Answer

Role of the Nurse Aide: Member of the Health Care Team

2. **The ombudsman is:**

   a. a client advocate.

   b. the state surveyor.

   c. a member of the clergy.

   d. in charge of the nursing home.

Answer

Role of the Nurse Aide: Member of the Health Care Team

3. **A member of the clergy is:**

   a. an employee of the activities department.

   b. a volunteer ombudsman.

   c. priest, rabbi, minister, or spiritual advisor.

   d. an administrative employee.

Answer

Role of the Nurse Aide: Member of the Health Care Team

4. **The individual responsible for the overall operation of the facility is the:**

   a. director of nursing.

   b. charge nurse.

   c. social worker.

   d. administrator.

Answer

ANSWER: a

Rationale:
The ombudsman is a client advocate who visits the nursing home periodically to speak on behalf of clients and resolve problems.

ANSWER: c

Rationale:
The charge nurse is the nurse aide's immediate supervisor, although the director of nursing is his or her department head.

ANSWER: d

Rationale:
Each facility has an administrator who is responsible for overall facility operations.

ANSWER: c

Rationale:
Members of the clergy are religious and spiritual authorities or advisors.

Role of the Nurse Aide: Member of the Health Care Team

5. **The nurse aide is responsible for:**

   a. the management of the nursing unit.

   b. providing personal and hygienic care to clients.

   c. telling others what to do.

   d. the client's day-to-day activities.

Answer ➡

Role of the Nurse Aide: Member of the Health Care Team

6. **Which of the following is not a nurse aide responsibility?**

   a. Giving medications.

   b. Bathing clients.

   c. Feeding clients.

   d. Dressing clients.

Answer ➡

Role of the Nurse Aide: Member of the Health Care Team

7. **The nurse aide is assigned to do a procedure for which he has not been trained. The procedure involves using an unfamiliar piece of equipment. The nurse aide should:**

   a. perform the procedure, because it is part of his assignment.

   b. do everything except the unfamiliar procedure.

   c. ask another nurse aide to care for the client.

   d. inform the nurse that he does not know how to perform the procedure.

Answer ➡

Role of the Nurse Aide: Member of the Health Care Team

8. **When reporting information to the supervisor, the nurse aide should report information that is:**

   a. subjective.

   b. personal.

   c. objective.

   d. confidential.

Answer ➡

ANSWER: a

Rationale:
Giving medications is not a nurse aide responsibility.

ANSWER: b

Rationale:
The nurse aide is responsible for providing personal and hygienic care to clients. The other choices listed here refer to jobs of other employees.

ANSWER: c

Rationale:
Objective information reflects things that you can see, feel, hear, or touch using your senses. Report information that is objective. Avoid subjective information that reflects your opinion. Do not disclose confidential information that has no bearing on the client's care.

ANSWER: d

Rationale:
The nurse aide should not perform procedures for which he has not been trained. He should inform the nurse that he is not familiar with the equipment and does not know how to perform the procedure.

Role of the Nurse Aide: Member of the Health Care Team

9. You overheard a coworker in the break room saying that you do not provide good care. The best way to handle this is to:

a. arrange to meet with the coworker to discuss the situation.

b. refuse to work with this individual.

c. ask the charge nurse to handle it.

d. tell the clients that the coworker is not a good nurse aide.

Answer ☛

Role of the Nurse Aide: Member of the Health Care Team

11. AIDS is the abbreviation for:

a. acquired immune deficiency syndrome.

b. isolation techniques.

c. a surgical procedure.

d. amputation of the arm.

Answer ☛

Role of the Nurse Aide: Member of the Health Care Team

10. HS care is given at:

a. breakfast.

b. lunch.

c. dinner.

d. bedtime.

Answer ☛

Role of the Nurse Aide: Member of the Health Care Team

12. Mr. Nielsen receives a nutritional supplement qd at 10 A.M. You know this means:

a. once a week at 10 A.M.

b. every day at 10 A.M.

c. three times a week at 10 A.M.

d. four times a day, with the first supplement given at 10 A.M.

Answer ☛

ANSWER: d

Rationale:
HS care is given at bedtime. HS is the abbreviation for "hour of sleep."

ANSWER: a

Rationale:
The best way to handle this situation is to meet with the coworker to discuss it and see if you can find common ground on which to agree. Avoid making remarks about the coworker to other clients and staff.

ANSWER: b

Rationale:
qd is the abbreviation for every day. Mr. Nielsen receives the supplement every day at 10 A.M.

ANSWER: a

Rationale:
AIDS is acquired immune deficiency syndrome, a serious condition spread by the human immunodeficiency virus (HIV).

Role of the Nurse Aide: Member of the Health Care Team

13. Mrs. Flotsan takes Tylenol PRN for pain. You know this means the client:

a. gets Tylenol every day.

b. may have Tylenol once a week.

c. may have Tylenol as needed for pain.

d. receives Tylenol routinely.

Answer ➜

Role of the Nurse Aide: Member of the Health Care Team

14. The nurse writes on your assignment to take Miss Hoyle's temp P.O. You know this means to:

a. keep the temperature warm in the client's room.

b. take the client's temperature by the axillary method.

c. avoid temperature extremes with this client.

d. take the client's temperature by mouth.

Answer ➜

Role of the Nurse Aide: Member of the Health Care Team

15. You are assigned to ambulate a client in the hallway. You know this means to:

a. walk the client in the hallway.

b. seat the client in a chair in the hall.

c. prevent the client from going into the hall.

d. push the client down the hall in a wheelchair.

Answer ➜

Role of the Nurse Aide: Member of the Health Care Team

16. Mr. Wells has a UTI. You know this is a:

a. cold.

b. urinary infection.

c. respiratory infection.

d. flu virus.

Answer ➜

ANSWER: d

Rationale:
PO is the abbreviation for "by mouth." In this case, the abbreviations mean you must take Miss Hoyle's temperature by mouth.

ANSWER: b

Rationale:
UTI is the abbreviation for "urinary tract infection."

ANSWER: c

Rationale:
PRN is the abbreviation for "as needed." Mrs. Flotsan may have Tylenol as needed for pain.

ANSWER: a

Rationale:
Ambulate means to walk. In this case, you will walk the client in the hallway.

Role of the Nurse Aide:
Member of the Health Care Team

17. The nurse writes on your assignment sheet to provide incontinent care for Mrs. Hernandez. You will give the client:

a. an enema.

b. a disposable brief.

c. perineal care.

d. a blue pad.

Answer ➜

Role of the Nurse Aide:
Member of the Health Care Team

18. You know that the terms bedsore and decubitus are sometimes used when referring to a:

a. skin tear.

b. bruise.

c. rash.

d. pressure ulcer.

Answer ➜

Role of the Nurse Aide:
Member of the Health Care Team

19. A set of symptoms affecting the client's thinking, judgment, and ability to reason is:

a. edema.

b. cyanosis.

c. anasarca.

d. dementia.

Answer ➜

Role of the Nurse Aide:
Member of the Health Care Team

20. The nurse assigns you to provide postmortem care. You know this means:

a. care of a client after death.

b. incontinent care.

c. after-meal care.

d. routine daily care.

Answer ➜

ANSWER: d

Rationale:
Bedsore and decubitus ulcer are sometimes used when referring to pressure ulcers.

ANSWER: a

Rationale:
Postmortem care is given to a client's body after death.

ANSWER: c

Rationale:
Perineal (peri) care is the same as incontinent care. The two terms are sometimes used interchangeably.

ANSWER: d

Rationale:
Dementia is a set of symptoms affecting thinking, judgment, and ability to reason. Dementia is a medical problem. Alzheimer's disease is the most common type of dementia.

Role of the Nurse Aide: Member of the Health Care Team

21. Mrs. McCloskey has an ecchymosis. You know that this is a/an:

a. laceration.

b. bruise.

c. rash.

d. edema.

Answer ➜

Role of the Nurse Aide: Member of the Health Care Team

22. The nurse aide knows that feces, stool, and

a. laceration are interchangeable terms.

b. edema are interchangeable terms.

c. bowel movement all mean the same thing.

d. urination all mean the same thing.

Answer ➜

Role of the Nurse Aide: Member of the Health Care Team

23. The nurse aide knows that an injury commonly caused by friction or shear is a/an:

a. abrasion.

b. bruise.

c. laceration.

d. cyanosis.

Answer ➜

Role of the Nurse Aide: Member of the Health Care Team

24. Mrs. Babitsky is NPO for a laboratory test. You know this means the client:

a. must stay in bed.

b. can have water, but not food.

c. can have food, but not water.

d. may have nothing by mouth.

Answer ➜

ANSWER: c

Rationale:
Feces, stool, and bowel movement all refer to waste products from the colon. The terms are often used interchangeably.

ANSWER: d

Rationale:
NPO is the abbreviation for "nothing by mouth." Mrs. Babitsky may not eat or drink anything.

ANSWER: b

Rationale:
Ecchymosis is the medical term for a bruise.

ANSWER: a

Rationale:
An abrasion is an injury commonly caused by friction or shear.

Role of the Nurse Aide: Member of the Health Care Team

25. Mr. Todd is on I&O. You know this means:

a. he must stay in his room.

b. his oral intake and fluid output must be measured.

c. he is in and out of bed ad lib.

d. his food intake must be monitored after each meal.

Answer ➔

Notes

Notes

Notes

Notes

ANSWER: b

Rationale:
I&O is the abbreviation for intake and output. Clients on I&O must have all fluid intake and output measured.